Common Scents

A Practical Guide to Aromatherapy

Lorrie Hargis

WOODLAND PUBLISHING
Pleasant Grove, Utah

The information in this book is for educational purposes only and is not recommended as a means of diagnosing or treating an illness. All matters concerning physical and mental health should be supervised by a health practitioner knowledgeable in treating that particular condition. Neither the publisher nor author directly or indirectly dispense medical advice, nor do they prescribe any remedies or assume any responsibility for those who choose to treat themselves.

Acknowledgments

This book could not have been possible without the support, inspiration and love of family, friends and clients given throughout the years.

A special thanks to Julie Detloff for her inspiration and drive, Nancy Jones for the work on developing the reflexology charts, Mary Fugitt for the endless hours of indexing, Nell Albitire for all the support, time and love, Patrick Collin for his willingness to help and answer any questions, Jack Ritchason for believing in me, Sarah Jones for the hours of typing, Mary Huston for enduring the long hours of putting everything together, Judy Evans for her perfection in editing this book, friendship and long hours, Jean Claude Pichot for his patience and support, my children, Burt and Danai, and parents Ben and Bonnie Hargis who have supported and loved me through it all. Thanks to all for making this possible.

There is an Indian proverb that says that everyone is a house with four rooms—a physical, a mental, an emotional and a spiritual. Most of us tend to live in one room most of the time, but unless we go into every room every day, even if only to keep it aired, we are not a complete person.

Contents

Foreword

I feel that whoever reads this book and puts to use the information that is in it will benefit both mentally and physically. Lorrie Hargis has proven herself to be one of the leading experts in the field of aromatherapy. She has been in the health field for many years working in the area of vitamins, minerals, and herbs. She certainly believes in touch therapy and is also greatly accomplished in emotional healing. I have known Lorrie for 15 years and found her to be very dedicated to any task she has undertaken. Her expertise in designing aromatic essential oil formulas has been proven. There have been many testimonials on Lorrie's formulas, her teaching abilities and her willingness to share this knowledge with others. She will not compromise her values by using inferior raw materials and will always search out the best. Lorrie is, and will always be, a person of integrity. We can look to Lorrie to always go after the most beneficial aspects of whatever endeavor she pursues.

Dr. Jack Ritchason

Introduction

My Goal

My goal in writing this book is to show how versatile aromatherapy is and how to use it with other natural healing modalities such as herbs, flower essences and treatments such as reflexology, acupressure, massage therapy and colonic therapy. My first child was born with a defect caused by Benedictine medication prescribed to me for morning sickness. She died 2 1/2 months later and I resolved to do my very best to raise any future children naturally. Realizing I had a choice was the answer.

Over the last 10 years I have had wonderful experiences using aromatherapy myself and sharing it with family, friends and clients. I am very happy to be able to share these experiences with you and hope you find them beneficial. Remember each of us are responsible for decisions concerning our health, and we have the free will to make these choices.

My Story

I became involved in aromatherapy and natural healing because of my desire to heal myself and my family. I was first introduced to natural healing through my mother.

My mother began having menopausal symptoms and read an article on foot reflexology in the local newspaper. She made an appointment with the reflexologist and purchased a foot/hand reflex chart and herbs and vitamins to support her reproductive system. After using the products, she started to see results; however, my father made fun of her and she stopped going to her appointments. He soon realized my mother had been benefiting from these reflexology treatments and nutritional supplements. In desperation, he found the reflexologist, and for Mother's Day he purchased gift certificates for my mom, sister and myself.

I went for my treatment and asked the reflexologist if she knew anyone who read eyes? She said, "Yes, I've been doing Iridology for ten years." I made an appointment for the following day to have my eyes read. After the reading, I began to follow the suggested regimen, which started me on a whole new life style. I followed the program she suggested, and within 6 weeks, I was losing weight and showed marked improvements in my health. My family and close friends noticed and began asking questions about the changes in my life. I felt healthy and renewed. I was on a mission to get my family healthy as well. I first decided to offer suggestions to my husband.

My husband had suffered with chronic allergies all his life. He would wake up and sneeze 50 times in the morning, cough all day, have headaches, and breathe heavily while resting. He was 28 years old and too young to have such health problems. He had become immune to all the over the counter (OTC) drugs for sinus and allergies. His poor health was very difficult on our relationship. He would come home from working a 12 hour day, eat very little, take a shower, turn the humidifier on, and go to sleep. His suffering was very hard on both of us. I knew something had to change. I also knew that each person makes their own personal decision to seek healing when they are ready.

My husband paid close attention to my improving health. Eventually, he asked me to take him to my herbalist. He decided that he wanted to become healthier. My herbalist told him the nutritional supplements that would strengthen his immune system. He followed her instructions and in three months he was starting to feel better.

As time went on and I developed a clientele, I began to utilize a small part of natural healing. One night, a client called extremely late and was emotionally upset. I tried to assure her if she took her herbs and B vitamins, she would be okay. She said, "You know herbs and vitamins aren't everything." I realized she was right, and I began a quest to study other modalities of natural health.

This led me to study flower essence therapy and become a practitioner. During this same time period, my family and I were at a local health food store. We discovered a book on aromatherapy and said, "Let's buy some of the essential oils that are mentioned in this book." We purchased lavender, clary sage, and geranium and started using the oils in our bath water. I noticed I had less difficulties with my premenstrual symptoms (PMS) when using the clary sage and geranium. Everyone's skin felt softer and had a glow to it.

Our son, Burt, had stuttered since age four. He often repeated words like ,"You see, you see, you see." This was extremely frustrating for him. From the ages of four to six, we took him to a speech pathologist for this stuttering problem. The pathologist said the school system would probably lose him between the cracks, because he most likely wouldn't qualify for help.

This is exactly what happened. I made many unsuccessful attempts to get him into a program. During fourth grade we changed schools and he was finally accepted into a speech therapy program but refused to go because he was embarrassed. When Burt was nine years old, we started putting five to ten drops of Lavender in his bath each night after reading that Lavender was calming. After one month, we all realized Burt was no longer stuttering. This convinced us to start experimenting with other essential oils. We used them in our baths, massage oils, lotions, shampoos, clay packs, facial steams and aroma lamps. We also successfully used the essential oils on our prize winning dairy goats, dogs and horses.

Then tragedy struck. Burt was ten years old when a 200-pound gate fell on his neck. This accident caused him to have constant headaches. My husband and I decided to go to some classes on orthobionomy to learn what we could do to stop Burt from having these horific headaches. We used the techniques we learned in class, along with essential oils and massage. Burt also had chiropractic treatments and kept his body built up with vitamins and herbs. Because of all of this, he was able to recover from the severe migraine headaches.

Aromatherapy then became my main focus. I started using different blends of essential oils for my client's challenges. I found essential oils

combined well with herbs, vitamins, flower essences, massage, orthobionomy and chiropractic. It seemed to be the spark that ignited people
to start healing. I believe aromatherapy is a healing modality that should
be used by everyone. I hope you will utilize the information in this book
to further your education in the use of essential oils to help enrich your
life and the lives of others around you.

History of Aromatherapy

In the 1920s, a chemist named René-Maurice Gattefossé rediscovered
the healing properties of aromatic essential oils in his family's perfumery. While working in the laboratory, Rene' was burned by an explo-
sion and immediately stuck his hand into a vat of Lavender oil. His hand
healed rapidly, with no infection or scarring. Rene' began studying the
medicinal properties of essential oils. He was the first person to describe
the use of these oils as "aromatherapy."

Essential oils help restore health and beauty. They relieve stress, and
tension, provide de-toxification for specific organs of the body, induce
deep relaxation, relieve muscle spasms and stimulate emotions of the
psyche.

Traditional healing practices have used aromatherapy for thousands of
years. Early man was the original researcher in this field. He gathered
roots, leaves and flowers as food, and accidentally discovered their healing properties when he applied them to his skin. This information was
passed down from generation to generation. Additionally, these people
burned trees and bushes, and the smoke gave off an aroma that made the
people feel differently. This smoking perfume was called incense. Wood
and resins from trees and bushes such as myrrh and frankincense were
burned to exalt the spirit.

Man soon began to travel and trade spices. With increasing ease and
speed of travel, they journeyed to new and unknown places for the first
time in history. People were exposed to new and different germs, viruses, and sexually transmitted diseases, and they turned to spices to help
combat these pathogens. The hotter spices, pepper, coriander, fennel,
cinnamon, and nutmeg, were found to have properties which aided in
digestion and helped fight pathogens.

As society became more sophisticated, they began discovering and using essential oils such as ylang ylang, patchouli, jasmine, vetiver, and sandalwood as perfumes to help mask body odors. In Persia, France, India, China, Babylon, and Egypt, essential oils were being used for medicinal purposes, embalming, holy anointing, and mummification.

Today, everyone can benefit from aromatherapy, an art traditionally reserved for kings and queens. We can utilize the collected knowledge of history and the latest scientific research to experience the finest aromatherapy products available and to help promote an age of healing and physical prosperity never known before.

What Is an Essential Oil?

Essential oils bring us the vital energies from the plant to help heal us on many levels: physically, emotionally, mentally and spiritually. These energies, stimulated by the sun and made active as the plant matures, are concentrated as well as subtle. The vapors are the subtle energies given off and absorbed by the cilia in the nose and mucous membranes. These vital energies come from the inside of roots, seeds, stems, leaves, flowers, wood bark, resins, and the peel of citrus fruits, and are extracted by different methods of distillation. Traveling through these mucous membranes, they reach the olfactory bulbs triggering the hypothalamus, which is located in the limbic part of the brain. Instincts, memories, and emotions of pleasure and pain are stored in this part of the brain. The hypothalamus then sends a message and the essential oil transports it wherever it is needed to balance the life force of the mind, body and soul.

Essential oils are used therapeutically in a natural health or healing modality called aromatherapy. Essential oils are therapeutic, because they have antiviral, antibacterial, anti-fungal, analgesic, calming, soothing and revitalizing chemical constituents. Each essential oil can be placed into a chemical family. There are many different chemical constituents to each essential oil. These chemical constituents are what give essential oils their many therapeutic qualities. For example, lavender is known to be antiviral, antibacterial, and to help calm, soothe and refresh you.

This is why using essential oils in your everyday life, only makes common sense/scents?

Essentials oils help with all kinds of physical ailments. An elderly client of mine has had arthritis and chronic pain for over thirty years. She also had a knee replacement about eight years ago. Essential oils of clove, nutmeg, and ginger, allow her to sleep at night without pain and keep her other knee mobile.

Essential oils can help balance emotions as well. During a class, a student came in late and was terribly distraught. She had been in a car wreck and could not stop crying. A drop of Geranium essential oil put on a cotton ball and held under her nose was able to calm her down so she could tell us what had happened. Smelling the vapors can balance us emotionally, as well as bring up memories from our subconscious. The first time I smelled cistus, I thought of my visits with my great grandmother in her living room.

At one time or another we all become confused, because we have too many things going on and become mentally stressed. Again, because of these many chemical constituents, an essential oil like peppermint, can help us to clear our minds with it's refreshing, cooling and stimulating aroma.

Spiritually, essential oils are a necessity. By balancing us physically, emotionally, and mentally, essential oils are going to help us spiritually. In all cultures from the beginning of time, aromatherapy is used in religious rituals. Frankincense is still used in churches during baptisms. It allows one to breathe deeply, clear your mind, and pray or meditate with clear intentions.

Chemical Families of Essential Oils

PHENOLS

Most of the properties of this chemical family are bactericidal with a large spectrum of action. These properties exist whether they are used internally or on the skin. Phenols kill parasites and have antifungal and antiviral properties. They stimulate the immune system. It is best when 3% (23 drops) of phenols are added to a carrier oil.

Contraindications: If you use phenols too long, they can suppress the immune system and can also cause hepatotoxicity. Phenols can become an irritant to the skin and the mucous membranes.

Examples of Essential Oils Containing Phenols: Clove (*Eugenia caryophyllata*), Oregano (*Origanum compactum*), Savory (*Satureja montana*), Thyme (*Thymus vulgaris C.T. thymol*).

TERPENES

Almost all essential oils contain some terpenes. Terpenes are good general tonics. They stimulate the cortico-surrenal glands which produce cortisone and this helps fight against pain and inflammation. When diffused into the air, terpenes are aerial antiseptics which do not eliminate bacteria but keep it from multiplying. They also stimulate the digestive, lymphatic and circulatory system.

Contraindications: Terpenes can cause the skin to dry out and to become thick. They can also cause irritation to the mucous membranes.

Examples of Essential Oils Containing Terpenes: Pine (*Pinus sylvestris*), Juniper (*Juniperus communis*), Lemon (*Citrus limonum*), Grapefruit (*Citrus paradisii*).

ALDEHYDES

Aldehydes are known for their anti-infectious, antifungal action. They are calming to the nervous system and powerful antiseptics when diffused. Aldehydes help to dissolve kidney stones and gallstones; they stimulate the liver and increase circulation to the skin. This makes them very beneficial for cellulite. Aldehydes are effective against herpes and are calming to type A, or easily stressed, personalities.

Contraindications: Aldehydes can be a skin irritant.

Examples of Essential Oils Containing Aldehydes: Eucalyptus (*Eucalyptus citriodora*), Lemongrass (*Cymbopogan citratus*) Lemon Verbena (*Lippia citriodora*).

KETONES

Essential oils high in ketones are antiviral, antifungal and protect the healthy cells from being infected by viruses and fungi. They can be helpful getting rid of warts and scars. Ketones assist in the digestion of fat and help move mucous out of the body via the bronchioles and the vagina.

Contraindications: Ketones are neuro-toxic and abortive.

Examples of Essential Oils Containing Ketones: Sage (*Salvia officinalis*), Hyssop (*Hyssopus officinalis*), Thuya (*Thuya occidentalis*).

*These contain less ketones and have more camphor which is less dangerous to the body: Rosemary (*Rosemary officinalis*, contraindicated in high blood pressure, epilepsy), Helichrysum (*Helichrysum italicum*), Dill (*Anethum gravoelens carvone*).

ESTERS

Esters are balancing, soothing, anti-spasmodic, anti-inflammatory and antibacterial. They also help to heal scars. Most are user friendly on the skin, and so are good for people who are hypertensive and stressed.

Examples of Essential Oils Containing Esters: Lavender (*Lavandula angustifolia*), Roman Chamomile (*Anthemis nobilis*), Ylang Ylang (*Canaga odorata*), Clary Sage (*Salvia sclarea*)

SESQUITERPENES

Sesquiterpenes are anti-inflammatory, anti-allergenic, bactericidal, antiseptic and calming.

Examples of Essential Oils Containing Sesquiterpenes: Yarrow (*Achillea illefolia*), German Chamomile (*Matricaria recutita*)

ETHERS

Oils containing ethers are anti-spasmodic for neuro and muscular disorders. They are anti-inflammatory, anti-allergenic and stimulating for individuals who are weak and depressed.

Examples of Essential Oils Containing Ethers: Tarragon (*Artemisia dracunculus ct. methlcharvicol*), Basil (*Ocium basilicum ct. methlcharvicol*), Fennel (*Foencullum vulgare*)

ALCOHOLS

Alcohols are strong bactericides, anti-infectious and antiviral. They are stimulating, warming and toning to the skin. Since these oils contain a high percentage of alcohol, they are regarded as good oils to use on children and the elderly. They seldom cause skin irritation.

Examples of Essential Oils Containing Alcohols: Sweet Thyme (*Thyme linolol*), Tea Tree (*Melaleuca alternifolia*), Geranium (*Pelargonium asperum*), Bergamot (*Citrus bergamia*; phototoxic), Neroli (*Citrus bigaradia*), Peppermint (*Mentha piperita*; do not use on children under 2), Palmaros (*Cymbopogen martini*)

Section 2

Applications

There are many pathways through which aromatherapy can travel into our bodies. This makes it one of the easiest forms of therapy to apply. No matter what the situation is, from the acute to the degenerative stage, aromatherapy can be helpful.

One of my clients who has been trying unsuccessfully for years to conceive a child using modern medicine said to me, "I've given up trying the medical route. People in the medical profession have forgotten that it's not the end that matters, but the journey there that counts."

After hearing her speak these words, I realized aromatherapy is a journey of its own and can help us on so many levels, no matter where our path is leading us. We might not completely cure someone of their disease; however, we will be able to ease their pain and suffering, and allow them to have a better quality of life in the present moment.

To make the effects of aromatherapy most beneficial it is important to understand the four stages of disease—acute, subacute, chronic and degenerative. Acute is when something suddenly comes upon us with sharp and severe pain, such as a toothache. It usually lasts for a short period of time(1 to 7 days). When treating acute conditions with aromatherapy, you can apply several different essential oils directly to the body with no carrier oil. Please refer to contraindications for each essential oil before direct (neat) application.

Subacute is where the acute situation continues on for 7 to 28 days. After 28 days the situation becomes chronic, and the body becomes more sluggish. The final stage, degenerative, is when the body completely loses the integrity of the tissue.

Some of the external pathways that can be beneficially combined with aromatherapy for acute, subacute, chronic and degenerative stages are sniffing ("the nose knows"), baths, sitz baths, colonics, clay packs, compresses, diffusions, inhalations, salves/ointments, acupressure, reflexology and massage. Do not use deep tissue massage in degenerative stage. Internal uses include gargling, ingesting orally, enemas, suppositories and douches.

When using aromatherapy's pathway of sniffing, take a test strip (Q-tip or strip of card stock) dip it carefully into one essential oil and gently move it in a clockwise motion under your nose. It is probably a good idea to test only 3 or 4 individual oils at a time to prevent confusion. To clear the aroma after each oil, sniff coffee beans, a wool garment or something else that will produce a similar effect. Select the oil that pleased you the most and try sniffing it during the day. It may help with headaches, nervous tension and emotional disturbances.

For example, one evening I was teaching a class when a woman walked in and said, "I have a terrible headache, I think I'll go home." I offered her lavender to sniff. She tried it and said, "Oh, that's awful." She then sniffed peppermint and said, "That's even worse." Finally, I took Blend#5 (Rosemary, Basil, Lavender, and Grapefruit) and let her sniff it. She said, "Yes, oh, my head feels better." Then she put a drop on each temple and on the back of her neck. Within a few minutes her headache was gone, and she did well throughout the rest of the class. Remember, "the nose knows." People know when an oil resonates with them. Sometimes they just need to be reminded to listen to themselves.

Solubol™

Solubol™ is a new and exciting product for aromatherapy users. It is a complex, vegetable emulsion that can be used internally (gargling, ingesting orally, enemas, and douches) and externally (baths, sitz baths, compresses, lotions). The ingredients are water, vegetable glycerin, soy lecithin, Rosemary extract, ascorbic acid, and vitamin E. Solubol™ is creamy and sweet tasting. It acts as the perfect carrier agent for essential oils and has a shelf life of two years. It must be kept at room temperature (68), protected from light, and kept dry (keep away from humidity). It is best to use the combination within a few hours, after diluting it with water or juice.

Internal Use of Solubol™

Solubol™ bypasses the stomach and goes directly to the small intestine, where it is readily absorbed in the body. It keeps the essential oils from irritating the mucous membranes. This is very important when using clove, cinnamon, oregano, and red thyme. These essential oils are in the phenol family, which contain carvacol and thymol, chemical components that are irritating to the mucous membranes.

SOLUBOL™ RECIPE FOR INFECTION IN ADULTS

50 drops Clove or Oregano or Blend #6 essential oils
1 T. Solubol ™
2 T. purified water (juice can be used)

For adults, always remember to use 8 times as much Solubol ™ as essential oil. For example, if a recipe calls for 9 drops essential oil(s), 72 drops of Solubol™ are needed (9x8). Squeeze Solubol™ into a glass, stir in essential oils and add water or juice. Drink ten drops three to six times daily.

SOLUBOL™ RECIPE FOR INFECTION IN CHILDREN(5-12 YEARS)

25 drops Sweet Thyme essential oil
1 T. plus 1 t. Solubol™
2 T. purified water (juice can be used)

For children, always remember to use 9 times as much Solubol ™ as essential oil. For example, if recipe calls for 10 drops of essential oil(s), 90 drops of Solubol™ are needed (10x9). Squeeze Solubol™ into a glass, stir in essential oil, and water or juice. Drink three to five drops three to six times daily.

Contraindications: Do not use essential oils internally with children under five or during pregnancy.

External Use of Solubol™

There are many wonderful ways to use Solubol™ externally. Essential oils and water do not mix, but when combined with Solubol™ will disperse easily into the water where the oils are readily absorbed by the skin. It can be used as a lotion when mixed with essential oils and applied directly on the skin.

SOLUBOL™ RECIPE FOR ADULT BATH

    10 drops essential oil
    1 t. (60 drops) Solubol ™

Squeeze Solubol™ into a small container. Add essential oil(s). Stir and add a little water to make it pour easily. Pour in as tub is filling.

SOLUBOL™ RECIPE FOR CHILDREN'S BATH: (CHILDREN 1-9 YRS)

    5 drops essential oil
    1/2 t. of Solubol™

Squeeze Solubol™ into a small container. Add essential oil(s). Stir and add a little water to make it pour easily. Pour in as tub is filling.

External Applications of Aromatherapy

Baths

There are two ways in which essential oils are transported into the body by a bath. First, by smelling the vapors that rise up from the warm water, and then when the pores in the skin open up and transport the essential oils into the blood stream. This makes it a valuable tool for all stages of disease. Baths are healing for all aspects of ourselves physically, emotionally, mentally and spiritually. A bath not only cleanses the body, but our minds as well.

GENERAL BATH RECIPE

> 10 to 15 drops essential oils(Lavender 1-5 drops for relaxation, 6-15 drops for balancing) or (Roman Chamomile 1-15 drops for calming) (Orange or Lemon 1-15 drops)
>
> 1 t. Solubol™ (not an essential ingredient, however, it makes essential oils much more effective).

Squeeze 1t. Solubol™ into a small container. Add essential oils and enough water to make it pour easily into tub as it is filling. Soak for at least 15 minutes, making sure you get all parts of your body wet with the wonderfully aromatic water. Turn on your sides and stomach, even go under the water if you like.

BATH RECIPE FOR BRUISING

> 5 drops Rosemary essential oil 5 drops Tea Tree essential oil
>
> 5 drops Helichrysum essential oil
>
> 1 t. Solubol™ (not an essential ingredient, however , it makes essential oils much more effective)
>
> 48 oz. apple cider vinegar

Squeeze 1 t. Solubol ™ into a small container. Add essential oils and enough water to make it pour easily. Add this Solubol™/essential oil blend to the apple cider vinegar and pour into tub as it is filling. Soak for at least 15 minutes. I put apple cider vinegar in my bath recipes because of its antiseptic, antibiotic, and pH balancing properties. It can be helpful when the hair and skin are too oily or too dry. It draws impurities out of the skin which makes it beneficial for blemishes, relieving arthritis, infection of the face, eyes, ears, cuts, and wounds.

BATH RECIPE FOR CHILLS, COLDS, FLUS AND NAUSEA

8 drops Blend #6 (Tea Tree, Ravensara, Lavender, Roman Chamomile essential oils)

2 drops Ginger essential oil

1 t. Solubol ™ (not an essential ingredient, however, it makes essential oils much more effective)

Squeeze 1 t. Solubol™ into a small container. Add essential oils and enough water to make it pour easily into tub as it is filling. Soak for at least 15 minutes, making sure you get all parts of body wet with the wonderfully aromatic water. Turn on your sides and stomach, even go under the water if you like.

BATH RECIPE FOR MENSTRUAL CRAMPS

9 drops Blend #3 (Clary Sage, Geranium, Rose Bulgarian, Nutmeg) essential oils

1 drop of Ginger essential oil

1 t. Solubol™ (not an essential ingredient, however, it makes essential oils much more effective)

Squeeze 1t. Solubol™ into a small container. Add essential oils and enough water to make it pour easily into tub as it is filling. Soak for at least 15 minutes, making sure you get all parts of body wet with the wonderfully aromatic water. Turn on your sides and stomach, even go under the water if you like.

BATH RECIPE FOR SINUS CONGESTION

5 drops Niaouli essential oil

4 drops Geranium essential oil

1 drop Ginger essential oil

1 t. Solubol ™ (not an essential ingredient; however, it makes essential oils much more effective)

Squeeze 1 t. Solubol™ into a small container. Add essential oils and enough water to make it pour easily into tub as it is filling. Soak for at least 15 minutes, making sure you get all parts of body wet with the wonderfully aromatic water. Turn on your sides and stomach, even go under the water if you like.

The above formulas for cold body conditions contain ginger because of its warming properties.

Sitz Bath

Sitz baths are used for the lower parts of the body. They are helpful for muscular pain, tension, hemorrhoids and after childbirth.

SITZ BATH RECIPE FOR AFTER CHILDBIRTH

1 qt. (32 oz.) boiling, distilled water

3 T. dried herbs of Comfrey or Marshmallow or 1 1/2 T. fresh herbs

20 drops Blend #7 (Roman Chamomile, Mandarin, Lavender, Rose essential oils)

20 drops Arnica flower essence

1 t. Solubol™ (not an essential ingredient, however, it makes essential oils much more effective)

To use this recipe you will first need to make an infusion (tea). Pour the quart of boiling water over the dried/fresh herbs and steep for 15 to 30 minutes. Make sure you cover with a lid as this keeps the volatile oils in the herbs. Plant leaves, stems and flowers are perfect for infusions. Use glazed earthenware, porcelain, porcelain lined or glass pots. An infusion can be kept in the refrigerator for up to a week, but should be used quickly because its medicinal properties decompose.

After finishing the infusion, mix Blend #7, flower essence and Solubol™ in a small container. Add the mixture into the infusion of comfrey or marshmallow and pour into a pan or partially filled tub. Soak for at least 15 minutes. If area is inflamed, use cool water for the Sitz bath.

SOOTHING AND CALMING BATH RECIPE FOR BABIES

1 drop Neroli essential oil

1 drop Lavender essential oil or 2 drops Blend #10 (Neroli, Geranium, Rose, Roman Chamomile, and Bergamot essential oil)

5 drops Chamomile flower essence

10 drops Solubol™ (not an essential ingredient, however, it makes essential oils much more effective)

Squeeze Solubol™ into a small container. Add essential oils, flower essence and enough water to make it pour easily into tub as it is filling. Soak for at least 5 minutes.

Clay

The healing properties of clay were popularized by the French Naturopath, Raymond Dextriet. Clay is known to help with the absorption, neutralizing and draining of the impurities in the body. It is beneficial for blemishes, wrinkles, insect bites, boils, abesses and inflammation caused by problems like sprains and arthritis.

Clay can be used cold, warm, or hot depending on the condition of the ailment. When used on a hot condition (stressed or overactive state) use cold clay. If after several minutes the afflicted area becomes too cold, remove the clay. If the area remains hot, remove and discard clay and make a new clay pack. Warm clay can be used to revitalize a cold condition (weakened or under active state) of the liver, kidneys, and gall bladder.

Contraindications for Clay : Wait at least 2 hours after eating before applying cold clay and one hour for hot clay. Remove clay packs one hour before eating. Do not use on lower abdomen during menstruation, unless there is a fever present. Do not apply in two different areas of the body at the same time. Throw clay away after application.

Important: When clay has dried and detached itself, it has completed its job.

CLAY RECIPE FOR SHINGLES

From personal experience, I have found that clay and aromatherapy help bring relief from the pain and swelling of shingles. This is the recipe that I found to be helpful.

Small bowl made of porcelain, enamel, wood, or glass
2 T. gray clay (Bentonite)
2 T. cold water
2 drops Tea Tree essential oil
2 drops Roman Chamomile essential oil
2 drops Geranium essential oil

Mix clay, water, and essential oils into a thick paste. Apply about 1/4" thick to the affected area. Apply new clay every 2 to 3 hours. When the heat and pain lessen, put on just once or twice a day. The eruptions will start drying up, and there will be less scarring.

CLAY RECIPE FOR BRUISES

2 drops Pine essential oil
2 drops Tea Tree essential oil
1 drops Rosemary essential oil
1 drop Peppermint essential oil
1 1/2 t. clay (Bentonite/Kaolin)
1 1/2 t. water

Mix clay, water and essential oils into a thick paste. Apply about 1/2" to 1" thick to the affected area. If the area is hairy, put a piece of cotton flannel cloth between the clay and hair. Leave on for 2 hours, unless the clay gets hot or dries quickly. Keep reapplying until the pain is gone.

CLAY RECIPE FOR SINUS CONGESTION AND PAIN

- 1 1/2 t. gray clay (Bentonite/Kaolin)
- 1 1/2 t. warm water
- 1 drops of Blend #1 (Niaouli, Rosemary, Geranium, and Peppermint) essential oils.

Mix clay, water, and Blend #1 into a thick paste. Apply about 1/4" thick to forehead and cheeks, keep away from eyes, as peppermint can irritate. Leave on until it dries and rinse off with warm water.

CLAY RECIPE FOR ARTHRITIS PAIN AND INFLAMMATION

- 2 T. gray clay (Bentonite)
- 2 T. cold water (may need a little more)
- 5 drops of Blend #2 (Niaouli, Juniper, Sweet Thyme, Geranium, Rosemary, Vetiver essential oils)

Mix clay, water, and Blend #2 into a thick paste. Apply about 1/2" thick to the inflamed area. Leave on 1 to 2 hours, until heat and pain subside and rinse with cool water.

CLAY RECIPE FOR ACNE (PIMPLES AND BLACKHEADS)

- 1 1/2 T. gray clay (Bentonite/Kaolin)
- 1 1/2 T. cold water
- 2 drops Lavender essential oil
- 1 drop Ylang Ylang essential oil
- 1 drop Geranium essential oil

Mix clay, water and essential oils into a thick paste. Apply about 1/4" thick to the whole face or affected area. Leave on until it dries and rinse with cool water.

My teenagers use clay and essential oils on their faces for pimples and blackheads. You can either use this formula for your whole face or cut the recipe in half and use it for that one "rocky mountain on your forehead", as my daughter would say.

Inhalation

Inhalation was very familiar to me as a child. If I had a head cold, my mother boiled vinegar over the stove and had me put a towel over my head and breathe the vapors. When my brother had croup, she steamed up the bathroom and had him inhale the steam.

Inhalations are good for sinus problems, hard dry coughs, and releasing impurities from the skin. Be extremely careful using inhalation with asthmatics, as hot steam often worsens the condition.

RECIPE FOR BRONCHITIS INHALATION
   5 drops Frankincense essential oil
   2 drops Niaouli essential oil
   3 drops Lemon essential oil
   2 C. water

Bring water to boil and pour into glass or stainless steel bowl. Add essential oils. Place towel over head and bowl, and breathe in the steam for 8 to 10 minutes.

Compresses

Compresses are helpful in acute and chronic conditions such as fevers, pain, inflammation of the joints, sprains, strains, constipation, boils and abscesses. Compresses can be applied cold, warm or hot. They can be made with water or a carrier oil. I prefer to use castor oil or olive oil.

Water Compress

COLD WATER COMPRESS RECIPE FOR SPRAINS
   10 drops Roman Chamomile essential oil
   10 drops Sweet Marjoram essential oil
   6 drops Cypress essential oil
   1 T. Solubol™
   1 C. cold water

Mix essential oils and Solubol™ together in a stainless steel bowl. Slowly add cold water and mix thoroughly. Wet cloth with solution and squeeze excess water back into the bowl. Wrap sprained/strained area and cover with a dry towel. Leave on 1/2 to 1 hour and reapply solution every two hours until the swelling goes down. An ice pack could be placed on the towel to further reduce swelling.

Carrier Oil Compress

Another way to apply a compress is with a carrier oil, which helps break up impurities and move them out of the body.

CARRIER OIL COMPRESS RECIPE FOR CONSTIPATION

5 drops Orange essential oil
5 drops Ginger essential oil
1 drop Clove essential oil
2 drops Nutmeg essential oil
1 C. of Olive oil or Castor oil

Warm the carrier oil in a medium sized, non-metallic pan, to body temperature (98.6 F). Add essential oils and blend well. Soak wool flannel in solution and squeeze excess oil back into the pan. Lay cloth on lower abdomen and cover with plastic wrap and a heating pad (low setting). Leave on until affected area feels warm. If the compress becomes too hot and you feel nauseated, discontinue use.

Contraindications: Do not use on a child under 5 or during pregnacy.

Diffusion

Diffusion is beneficial as an expectorant and also as an inhalant to disperse vapors inside the lungs. In addition, it has the power to keep bacteria from multiplying and to create a pleasant environment.

In dispersing essential oils, a diffuser is more effective than an aromatherapy lamp. A diffuser disperses all the components of the essential oils at once; whereas, an aromatherapy lamp fractures and oxidizes a large portion of the essential oil by overheating.

I had an experience with diffusion when my daughter decided to have a party for some little girls. Several of them did not seem to get along. I told her she was silly to invite such enemies for a party together. She was really set on inviting these friends, so before the girls arrived I made a blend of Geranium, Palma Rosa, and Lemon essential oils. The party was a great success. I have also used this same blend for holidays with relatives to add a calming atmosphere.

DIFFUSER RECIPE FOR SOCIAL GATHERINGS
10 drops Geranium essential oil
10 drops Lemon essential oil
5 drops Palma Rosa or Bois de Rose essential oil
Place essential oils in glass nebulizer and operate diffuser according to manufacturers instructions.

How to clean after use: remove the glass nebulizer from the diffuser and clean with warm soapy water or rubbing alcohol. Do this before adding a new oil.

* Do not use massage oil or essential oils such as Vetiver, Jasmine, or Ylang Ylang in a diffuser, they are too thick.

Ointments/Salves

Ointments are usually made with olive oil, herbs and essential oils. You can make different kinds of ointments once you have prepared the base. Add tea tree oil for an antiseptic salve, peppermint for sore aching muscles, and eucalyptus for a decongestant. Ointments have been used for centuries to draw impurities out of the body, help heal wounds, cuts, burns, and soothe or beautify dry, chaffed skin.

OINTMENT RECIPE FOR HEALING SKIN
(Before making the ointment, an herbal oil infusion needs to be prepared)

HERBAL OIL INFUSION RECIPE
1/4 C. dried Comfrey leaves
1/2 C. dried Yarrow flowers
1 C. dried Lavender flowers
1/3 C. dried Roman Chamomile flowers
1 C. dried German Chamomile flowers
1 C. dried Calendula flowers
5-7 C. Olive oil
muslin cloth
large strainer
glass jar (2 quarts or larger)
large glass/crockery mixing bowl

Grind dried herbs into a fine powder using a mortar and pestle or blender. Place ground herbs in jar that can be capped tightly and add olive oil to cover the herbs. Stir the mixture well. After the herbs are wet, add more oil to cover the herbs an additional 1/4 to 1/2 inch, as some herbs will absorb this extra oil. Check the mixture 24 hours later to see if more oil needs to be added. Cap jar tightly, place it in a thick paper bag or box, to keep the light out, and place the box in the sun. Shake the mixture daily.

After 7 to 10 days, strain the oil from the herb by pouring the oil through a muslin cloth draped inside a strainer resting over a large glass bowl. This will take some time because the mixture is thick. When strained, gently press the pulp. Do not use too much pressure or small pieces of herbs will reenter the oil. Use a second piece of muslin and re-strain the oil. Pour infused oil in dark colored bottles, cap tightly, label, and store in a cool place.

OINTMENT RECIPE FOR WOUNDS, BITES, CUTS, AND SKIN DISORDERS
6 oz. Beeswax
120 drops Blend #6 essential oils or 50 drops Tea Tree essential oil,
50 drops Roman Chamomile essential oil
20 drops Lavender essential oil
Herbal oil infusion (from previous recipe)
Large glass pan

Small glass pan
Glass candy thermometer
Small ladle

Heat beeswax until melted in a small glass pan. It may take up to 140 degrees to melt. Be careful not to overheat, or wax will start to darken. While the beeswax is melting, warm the herbal oil infusion to 120 degrees. Remove the beeswax from the heat, and immediately begin slowly pouring into the oil infusion while stirring constantly. Then stir in essential oils. Make a test sample by taking a spoonful of your ointment and pouring onto a piece of wax paper. It should harden quickly. Feel to see if it's fairly creamy and will spread easily. Keep in mind, ointments are effected by body and environmental temperatures. You can always add more beeswax if you want a harder consistency; however, you will not be able to make it softer. Ladle ointment into glass jars. Don't move the jars or the ointment might crack or puddle. When ointment is cool, tightly screw lids on and label.

Ready-Made Ointments/Salves

It is more convenient to purchase a ready-made ointment and add essential oils to it. Ointment #11 contains Olive oil, Golden Seal Root, Yarrow Flowers, White Oak Bark, Black Walnut, Marshmallow Root, Lobelia, Scullcap, Myrrh Gum, Mullein, Wheat Germ, Chickweed, beeswax, Eucalyptus, and Vitamin E . This can be used for dry skin, cuts and wounds.

OINTMENT RECIPE FOR ANTISEPTIC PURPOSES
1oz. Salve #11
20 drops Blend #6(Tea Tree, Lavender, Ravensara, Roman Chamomile)

Add essential oils to ointment and mix thoroughly. Apply to affected area.

OINTMENT RECIPE FOR DRY, SCARRED, CRACKED, CHAPPED SKIN
1oz. Salve #11
20 drops Blend #7 (Roman Chamomile, Mandarin, Lavender, and Rose)

Add essential oils to ointment and mix thoroughly. Apply to affected area.

Drawing Ointment
Another ointment, #12, contains Olive oil, Chaparral Herb, Lobelia Herb, Comfrey Leaf, Marshmallow, Chickweed, Myrrh Gum, beeswax, Pine Tar, and vitamin E oil. This can be used to draw impurities from the body.

OINTMENT RECIPE FOR BOILS AND ABSCESSES
1oz. Ointment #12
20 drops Red Thyme (Sweet Thyme may be used, but takes longer)

Add essential oils to ointment and mix thoroughly. Apply to affected area.

Internal Applications of Aromatherapy

Suppositories

Suppositories are cylinders made with cocoa butter, herbs and essential oils, which are inserted into the rectum or vagina for therapeutic purposes. They liquefy at body temperature. Once the suppository has melted, the action of the essential oils and herbs passes into the veins in the lining of the anus, rectum or vagina and go directly into the blood stream.

Vaginal suppositories
Suppositories work well for vaginal infections, cancer of the cervix and endometrial cancer.

SUPPOSITORY RECIPE FOR VAGINAL INFECTION

20 capsules Chickweed
15 capsules Slippery Elm
15 capsules Yellow Dock
10 capsules Golden Seal Root
5 capsules Mullein Leaves
5 capsules Marshmallow Root
40 drops Tea Tree essential oil
60 drops Myrrh essential oil
20 drops Lavender essential oil
3oz. Cocoa Butter

Mix herbs together. Melt cocoa butter in a double boiler, add herbs and essential oils to make a thick, dough-like consistency. Cool sufficiently for handling. Roll small, finger sized cylinders, put on wax paper. If it's too wet when you make the suppositories, they will turn into flat flying saucers. Add more herbs. If it's too dry, add more cocoa butter. Let harden and refrigerate.

Put the suppositories in at night. You might need to wear a sanitary napkin. Leave in all day, then douche in the evening. Do this procedure for seven days .

Rectal Suppositories

Rectal suppositories are used for bronchial, lung infections, and prostatitis.

SUPPOSITORY RECIPE FOR ACUTE PROSTATITIS

100 drops Roman Chamomile essential oil
75 drops Lemon essential oil
40 drops Juniper essential oil
3oz. Cocoa Butter

Melt cocoa butter in double boiler and add essential oils to dough-like consistency. Cool sufficiently for handling. Roll small finger sized cylinders and place them on wax paper. Let harden and refrigerate. Coat with olive oil or coconut oil. Insert in the rectum three times daily for ten days.

SUPPOSITORY RECIPE FOR BRONCHIAL INFECTION (FOR ADULTS)

20 drops Ravensara
20 drops Lavender
20 drops Sweet Thyme
75 drops Niaouli or 125 drops of Blend #6(Tea Tree, Ravensara, Roman Chamomile, Lavender)
3oz. Cocoa Butter

Melt cocoa butter, add essential oils, let cool, and make into finger sized cylinders. Refrigerate. Insert in the rectum three times daily for ten days.

Enema

An Enema is the introduction of a liquid into the rectum and colon through the anus. Enemas are used to help with constipation, colds, flu, bronchial infections, and pain. This form of application is efficient and rapid.

COLD, FLU, AND INFECTION ENEMA RECIPE

4 drops Roman Chamomile essential oil
6 drops Eucalyptus Globulus essential oil
6 drops Tea Tree essential oil
1 qt. warm water
1 t. (2 ml) Solubol ™
3 Acidophilus or Bifidophilus Capsules
K-Y Jelly or Aloe Vera Gel
small glass bowl to position under enema bag

Warm purified water to body temperature. Put a towel on the floor and make sure the room is warm. Mix essential oils with the Solubol™ and add it to the warm water. Put water in the enema bag and hang the bag 36"off the floor. Set small glass bowl on floor under enema bag. Lie on your back and massage colon in a clockwise motion, from right to left with a carrier oil, or a blend from the Constipation Compress Recipe, to begin breaking up fecal matter. Get on your hands and knees. Slowly open the nozzle and let some water into the bowl to release any air in the tube. Check the temperature and flow of the water. Put K-Y Jelly or Aloe Vera Gel on the speculum and your rectum. Insert the lubricated speculum into the rectum, open the nozzle and let the water flow in. When you feel full turn off nozzle and excrete into the toilet. Sometimes it's best to release only about one cup of water at a time into the rectum and try to retain it for five minutes. This breaks up the fecal matter more readily. When finished, insert acidophilus and bifidophilus capsules coated with K-Y jelly or aloe vera gel into the rectum to replace beneficial intestinal flora.

*Do not use eucalyptus on asthmatics or children under two.

RECIPE FOR INFLAMMATION OF THE COLON ENEMA

10 capsules of Herbal Combination #13 (Slippery Elm Bark, Marshmallow Root, Plantain herbs, Chamomile flowers, Rosehips, and Bugleweed)
5 drops Roman Chamomile essential oil
5 drops Lemon essential oil
1t. Solubol ™
1qt. warm water
3 Acidophilus capsules
K-Y Jelly or Aloe Vera Gel
a small glass bowl to position under enema bag

Lie on your back and massage colon in a clockwise motion from right to left with a carrier oil, or a blend from the Constipation Compress Recipe, to begin breaking up fecal matter. Get on your hands and knees. Slowly open the nozzle and let some water into the bowl to release any air in the tube. Check the temperature, and the flow of the water. Put K-Y jelly or aloe vera gel on the speculum and your rectum. Insert the lubricated speculum into the rectum, open the nozzle and let the water flow in. When you feel full turn off nozzle and excrete into the toilet. Sometimes it's best to release only about one cup of water at a time into the rectum and try to retain it for five minutes. This breaks up the fecal matter more readily. When finished, insert acidophilus and bifidophilus capsules coated with K-Y jelly or aloe vera gel into the rectum to replace beneficial intestinal flora.

Section 3

Flower Essences

Flower essence and aromatherapy make a great partnership in balancing the mind, soul and body. Flower essences work first on the subtle energies, then the physical body. Aromatherapy goes first, to the subconscious and the physical body, then on to the subtle energies.

Flower essences were developed and pioneered by Dr. Edward Bach in the 1930's. Through his practice, he realized people couldn't get well when they were consumed with negative emotions. He believed when we rid ourselves of negative emotions, we are truly balanced. Dr. Bach felt he might find answers in nature and began to study plants and find their signatures. This work led him to develop 39 flower remedies. He found that flower essences are a very subtle healing modality. Each flower essence seemed to bring out a positive aspect of the personality.

The traditional way to use flower essence was under the tongue. Dr. Bach also spoke of using flower essences in compresses. Today, people are using them under the tongue, in the bath, for massage, in clay packs, compresses, and directly on the skin.

Case #1

For example, when we were leaving my mother's home, my six year old daughter slammed the car door on her toe. Immediately, I asked my mother to go and get her "Rescue Remedy" from the house. We applied the remedy directly on the toe. It not only took the emotional shock away, but the toe did not swell, or turn black and blue.

Case#2

A few years later, my mother and I were playing doubles with my daughter and her friend in a game of badminton. As my mother attempted to hit the birdie, her ankle completely rotated, and she fell in pain. I heard her ankle crack. I held her ankle still and told her to take deep breaths. My father put ice on her ankle while I drove home and got the "Rescue Remedy", which I mixed into a blend of essential oils of sweet marjoram, Roman chamomile, and cypress. We gently applied this mixture to her ankle while continuing to use the ice. My father took her to emergency to have the ankle x-rayed. Because of a previous experience of a horse breaking my three toes on my left foot and having my X-rays misread, I cautioned my mother to make sure that at least two people read her X-rays.

That evening I called to find out the test results. The lab technician said her ankle was just badly sprained. I felt this was not true, so we continued to put the flower remedy blend and ice packs on her ankle. The next morning, my father called my brother-in-law, who is a physical therapist, and asked his advice. He suggested that we get an air cast for her ankle, and that we alternate cold packs and heat therapy in the hot tub. He also gave her ankle exercises to do at home. With his program, she also continued to use her flower blend with a regimen of calcium, magnesium, B-Complex, and citrus bioflavonoids. Within two weeks her ankle was fine.

The ironical thing is that two weeks later, someone from the lab called and said, "Mrs. Hargis, we went over your x-rays again and found a fracture in your ankle." She said, "Oh, well my ankle is completely healed, thanks to my children's advice." Fortunately, my mother has never had any recurring weakness in her ankle.

This demonstrates how several modalities can compliment each other in healing. Dr. Bach wrote in the *Twelve Healers* that, "For pain, stiffness, inflammation, or any kind of local ailments one should also use a lotion.

A few drops from the stock bottle are put into a bowl of water and a piece of cloth is soaked in it and applied to the affected areas. If necessary one can rewet the cloth again and again."

Case#3

In another situation my husband came home for lunch. I went into the kitchen to speak to him and he wasn't there, but I could hear him moaning with pain in the living room. I ran in only to find him pouring with sweat and in severe pain. He was holding his lower abdomen. To find out what was wrong, I asked if he had been having problems urinating or eliminating from his bowels. He said they were fine. I remembered Dr. Jack Ritchason telling me when a man has pain all over his body for no apparent reason and his stools are the size of a pinkie finger, it could be acute prostatitis.

I put him into the bath tub with a blend of lavender, Roman chamomile essential oils and the "Rescue Remedy". He stayed in the bath tub for about 20 minutes. I couldn't give him anything orally because he thought he might throw it up. I put him in bed and applied ozonated olive oil to his lower abdomen. Then I slightly heated a combination of olive oil infused with dandelion herb, mixed with chamomile, lemon, juniper essential oils and a liquid herbal extract containing Valerian root, anise seed, black walnut hulls, desert tea herb, ginger root, and licorice root. I soaked the wool flannel in the mixture and applied it to his lower abdomen, followed by a piece of plastic wrap and a heating pad.

His pain and nausea started to subside, and he felt he was ready to take something internally. I mixed Roman chamomile, lemon, juniper essential oils and the "Rescue Remedy" into the Solubol™ for him to drink. After about an hour, he had to go to the bathroom. When he urinated he had severe pain as the prostate was swollen.

After another hour, the pain had subsided and he seemed to be over the attack. Within two hours, he came to my office door completely dressed and ready to go back to work. I said, "Are you sure you can go back to work?" "Oh yes, I'm fine," he responded. He left for work and I continued working in my office. Two hours later my daughter picked up the phone, and someone said they were dying. She became extremely upset, so I grabbed the phone. It was my husband. He had had another attack.

My son and I drove to where my husband was working and had to actually lift him off the seat of his truck into my car. I drove him home, got him back into the bath tub and went through the same procedure again. This time he took double doses of everything. By mid-evening, his pain had ceased. It took him two more days of taking the "Rescue Remedy" and Solubol™ with Roman chamomile, lemon and juniper essential oils, as well as zinc, saw palmetto, vitamin E, and citrus bioflavonoids, but he made a full recover. These are some true cases using flower essences and aromatherapy together.

Applications with Flower Essences and Aromatherapy

Now let's take a look at the different ways to use these two modalities together. First of all, have some kind of resource material for flower essences. I would suggest the Flower Essence Repertory by Patricia Kamanski and Richard Katz.

Read through the resource material and pick out just 4 or 5 different flower essences that you find interesting. Start using them either one by one or combined. Pick an essential oil with which you would like to take a bath, spritzer, or massage. Here are some suggestions you might like to try.

RECIPE FOR DETOXIFICATION BATH
1 qt. apple cider vinegar
10 drops *Blend #2 (Juniper, Sweet Thyme, Vetiver, Cypress, Grapefruit, Geranium).
1 t. Solubol™(refer to bath recipe)
5 drops Crab Apple flower essence
5 drops Self Heal flower essence
5 drops Chaparral flower essence
5 drops Yarrow flower essence

Mix essential oils and flower essences in with the Apple Cider vinegar and add it to the bath water. Squeeze 1 t. Solubol™ into a small container, add flower essences and essential oils and stir. Add a little water to make it pour more easily and pour into filled tub. Soak for at least 15 minutes.

HEMORRHOIDS SITZ BATH RECIPE
A sitz bath is great for relieving hemorrhoids, strained and tired muscles, and after giving birth.

2 drops Peppermint essential oil
5 drops Geranium essential oil
5 drops Cypress essential oil
10 drops Crab Apple flower essence
10 drops Self Heal flower essence
1 t. Solubol™

Pour the flower essences and essential oils in warm bath water. Squeeze 1 t. Solubol™ into a small container, add flower essences and essential oils, stir and add a little water to make it pour more easily. Pour into a filled tub. Soak for 15 minutes.

SPRITZER TENSION RELEASER RECIPE
Great for changing an environment or adding pleasant aroma to the room, whether that be relaxing, invigorating, romantic, or antibacterial.

2 oz. dark colored bottle with sprayer
15 drops of Lavender essential oil
7 drops of Grapefruit essential oil
7 drops of Ylang Ylang essential oil
10 drops Chamomile flower essence
10 drops Lavender flower essence

Mix essential oils and flower essences together. Add a little water to make it pour easily into the bottle. Finish filling bottle with water and shake well. Spray as needed.

MASSAGE OIL RECIPE TO ASSIST CONCENTRATION
2 oz bottle
30 drops Blend #5 (Rosemary, Basil, Grapefruit and Lavender)
5 drops Peppermint flower essence
5 drops Madia flower essence
5 drops Rabbitbrush flower essence
5 drops Self Heal flower essence
2 oz. massage oil

Pour essential oil blend, massage oil, and flower essences into the bottle. Roll the bottle back and forth to mix the contents together. Apply twice daily or as needed to temples, forehead, back of neck, brain and corresponding reflex points on the feet.

Compresses

Compresses help with inflammation and pain. They are soothing to the body and can help draw out impurities. Warm 1 oz. of carrier oil in a small pan on the stove. Add 15 drops of an essential oil combination or a single oil, and 20 drops of flower essences. Soak wool flannel in the mixture and lay over inflamed area, cover with plastic wrap and a heating pad on low setting. Leave in place until the affected area feels warm. You may feel nauseated if the compress becomes too hot. Discontinue use if this is the case. The most helpful compress carrier oils are herbal infused olive oil and castor oil. Oils such as almond and apricot can also be used.

Contraindication: Do not use during pregnancy.

CONSTIPATION COMPRESS RECIPE
1 oz. warmed olive oil
5 drops Peppermint essential oil
10 drops Rosemary essential oil
5 drops Orange essential oil
5 drops Crab Apple flower essence

5 drops Dandelion flower essence
5 drops Rock Rose flower essence
5 drops Self-Heal flower essence

Combine oils and essences. Soak wool flannel in mixture and place on lower abdomen. Cover with plastic wrap and a heating pad on low setting. Compress may take 10 minutes or so to warm the area. This same formula can also be used to massage the colon area before a colonic or enema.

CLAY PACK RECIPE
Beneficial for drawing out the impurities from boils, pimples, blackheads and whiteheads, constipation, and insect bites. They can also relieve hardened areas of the body. Clay packs will draw poisons out of the body and reduce inflammation.

Put 1 T. of clay in a small bowl. Add 5 drops of essential oil or blend, 1 1/2 t. of water and 10 drops of flower essences. Mix well. Consistency should be wet and thick. Smooth over affected area and let dry until clay cracks. Rinse off with cool water. Reapply clay pack if needed.

CLAY PACK RECIPE FOR SPRAINS, STRAINS, SWELLING OF MUSCLES
1 T. of clay
10 drops Roman Chamomile essential oil
10 drops Sweet Marjoram essential oil
20 drops Arnica flower essences
6 drops Cypress essential oil

Combine ingredients in a small bowl with 1 T. of cold water. Blend well. Consistency should be wet and thick. Place the clay pack on injured area and let dry until the clay cracks. Keep reapplying until the inflammation has gone down.

Enemas

BRONCHIAL INFECTION ENEMA RECIPE

1 qt. warm, purified water
5 drops Red Thyme essential oil
2 drops Niaouli essential oil
1 drop Ravensara essential oil
2 drops Frankincense essential oil
1 t. Solubol™
10 drops Yerba Santa flower essence
10 drops Self Heal flower essence
3 capsules of Acidophilus or Bifidophilus

Put a towel on the floor and make sure the room is warm. Lie on your back and massage your colon in a clockwise motion from right to left to relax the area and to help break up fecal matter. Use purified water heated to body temperature. Make sure you use K-Y jelly or aloe vera gel on your speculum. Hang the enema bag 36" off the floor. Mix essential oils and flower essences together in Solubol™ and combine with warm water. Get on your hands and knees. Slowly open nozzle and let some water into a bowl to release any air in the tube. Check temperature and flow of water. Insert lubricated speculum into the rectum. Open nozzle and let the water flow in. When you feel full, turn off nozzle, remove speculum and excrete into the toilet.

Sometimes it's best to only release about a cup of water into the rectum at a time and try to hold it for 5 minutes. This breaks up the fecal matter more readily. When finished, to replace beneficial intestinal flora, insert bifidophilus or acidophilus capsules coated with K-Y jelly or aloe vera gel.

Suggestions for Colonic Therapist

COLONICS

1.Use a blend of essential oils and flower essences to spritz the room before the client comes in, to help relax the patient and eliminate odors.

2. Massage the colon with the constipation compress recipe before and during the colonic to help break up fecal matter.

SPRITZER RECIPE FOR RELAXATION

25 drops Blend #10 (Neroli, Bergamot, Roman Chamomile, Rose, Bulgaria, Geranium)
20 drops Dandelion flower essence
20 drops Chamomile flower essence
2 oz. of water

Mix essential oils and flower essences together. Add water and put into sprayer with 2 oz. of water (1/4 cup). Shake well and spritz.

Douches

This procedure has been around a long time for women. Thirty years ago, it was very popular to douche. When I was growing up as a young woman, we were told not to douche, because it would destroy the pH balance of the vagina.

I believe that balance is very important in all things. If one is constantly having yeast infections, douching can be beneficial if not done more than once or twice a week.

DOUCHE RECIPE FOR YEAST INFECTIONS

1 qt. warm, purified water
5 drops Easter Lily flower essence
5 drops Pine flower essence
6 drops Myrrh essential oil
4 drops Lavender essential oil
4 drops Tea Tree essential oil
1 cup Apple Cider vinegar
2 Acidophilus or Bifidophilus capsules
1 t. Solubol™ (This is not an essential ingredient, however, it makes essential oils much more effective)

Squeeze 1 t. Solubol™ into a small container. Add flower essences, essential oils, Bifidophilus or Acidophilus capsules, stir and slowly add Apple Cider vinegar. Pour solution into douche bag. Put K-Y Jelly or Aloe Vera Gel on speculum. Insert tip and gently squeeze solution into vagina.

SUPPOSITORY RECIPE FOR ENDOMETROSIS
  2 oz. of Cocoa Butter
  10 drops Blend #3 (Clary Sage, Nutmeg, Rose, and Geranium)
  5 drops Black Cohosh flower essence
  5 drops Alpine Lily flower essence
  5 drops Self Heal flower essence
  5 drops Love-lies-Bleeding flower essence
  Herbal Formula Quing Re #14
  2 capsules of garlic herb

Melt Cocoa Butter in a double boiler. After the butter is melted add herbs, Blend #3 and flower essences. Mix thoroughly. Let cool, then roll the mixture into about 10 finger-sized boluses. Refrigerate boluses for 1 hour to make insertion easier. Before bed, while in a sitting position, insert bolus into vagina. Leave in until next evening. Then douche with the above recipe or 1 cup apple cider vinegar to 1 qt. of warm water. Insert new bolus. Repeat this procedure for 1 week. Extra boluses can be stored in refrigerator or freezer. **Note:** this is more frequent douching than normally recommended.

Section 4
Single Essential Oils

Basil

(Ocimum basilicum l. folium)
COUNTRY OF ORIGIN: Vietnam, France, Madagascar
LABIATAE FAMILY
It combines well with Rosemary, Peppermint, Lavender, Bergamot, Clary Sage, Geranium, Neroli and Frankincense.

Major Chemical Constituents: methylchavicol.

The aroma is hot, pungent and licorice-like. Basil is steam distilled. The parts used for extracting the essence are the leaves and flowering tops.

Circulatory System: Toning and stimulating to the circulation. *External Use:* Massage, bath, acupressure , reflexology.
Digestive System: Aids in digestion. *Internal Use:* Orally 3 to 5 drops in Solubol™ with water twice daily.
Glandular System: Helps tone and restore balance to the adrenals. *External Use:* Massage, reflexology, acupressure.
Immune System: Fevers, whooping cough. *External Use:* Massage, diffuse.

Intestinal System: Parasites, spasms of the intestine, antiseptic for the intestines, anti- bacterial. *Internal Use:* Orally 3 to 5 drops in Solubol™ with water twice daily.

Mind System: Mental fatigue, anxiet, depression, lack of energy, tiredness, confusion, fear, memory loss. *External Use:* Diffuse, massage, reflexology.

Nervous System: Headaches, migraines, anxiety, no energy. *External Use:* Massage, diffuse, compress. *Internal Use:* Orally 3 to 5 drops in Solubol™ with water twice daily.

Reproductive System: Menstrual difficulties such as pain and scanty or nonexistent periods. *Internal Use:* Orally 3 to 5 drops in Solubol™ with water three times daily.

Respiratory System: Expectorant, whooping cough, bronchitis, sinus. *External Use:* Diffuse, massage, reflexology, compress. *Internal Use:* Orally 3 to 5 drops in Solubol™ with water.

Skeletal System: Joint pain. *External Use:* Massage, reflexology, acupressure, compress.

Skin System: Draws out poison from insect bites, oily skin. *External Use:* Compress, clay pack.

Contraindications: Do not use during pregnancy.

Bergamot

(Citrus bergamia)
COUNTRY OF ORIGIN: Calabria, Italy
RUTACEAE FAMILY

It combines well with Bay, Black Pepper, Cardamon, Coriander, Ginger, Lemon, Grapefruit, Jasmine, Marjoram, Niaouli, Nutmeg, Orange, Patchouli, Palmarosa, Sandalwood, Vetiver and Ylang Ylang.

Major Chemical Constituents: linalool, limonene, linalyle acetate.

The aroma is refreshing, citrus-like, sweet and flowery. Bergamot's rind is cold pressed and it is the part used to extract the essence. The color is green to olive green.

Digestive System: Anorexia, stimulates appetite and digestion. *External Use:* Diffuse, bath, massage. *Internal Use:* Orally 3 to 5 drops in Solubol™ with water three times daily.

\Immune System: Chicken pox, herpes, antibiotic, cold, flu, fever. *External Use:* Massage. *Internal Use:* Orally 3 to 5 drops in Solubol™ with water three times daily.

Intestinal System: Intestinal parasites, laxative, colic. *Internal Use:* Orally 3 to 5 drops in Solubol™ with water twice daily.

Nervous System: Shingles, herpes, antispasmodic, insomnia, tiredness. *External Use:* Massage, bath, diffuse.

Mind System: Depression, anxiety, ,stress, tension, hysteria, emotional crisis, irritability, tiredness. *External Use:* Diffuse, bath, massage.

Reproductive System: P.M.S., vaginal itching. *Internal Use:* Douche.

Skin System: Oily skin balancing, psoriasis. *External Use:* Facials, massage, bath, ointment.

Urinary System: Kidney infection, disinfectant of the urinary tract. *Internal Use:* Orally 3 to 5 drops in Solubol™ with water three times daily.

Contraindication: Phototoxic.

Black Pepper

(Piper nigrum)
COUNTRY OF ORIGIN: Madagascar
PIPERACEAE FAMILY

It combines well with Vetiver, Frankincense, Clove, Jasmine, Lavender, Geranium, Rose, Ylang Ylang, Rosemary, Sandalwood, Orange, Lemon, Bergamot, Tea Tree, Fennel, Cardamon, Cinnamon, Coriander, Ginger and Nutmeg.

Major Chemical Constituents: α pinene, β pinene, D3 carene, limonene, β caryophyllene.

The aroma is warm, spicy, smooth, of fresh ground pepper. Black pepper is steam distilled. The part used in the extracting of the essence is the peppercorns. Black pepper is colorless.

Circulatory System: Stimulates circulation. *External Use:* Massage.

Digestive System: Calming to the stomach. *External Use:* Massage. *Internal Use:* Orally 3 to 5 drops in Solubol™ with water.

Immune System: Anti-microbial. *External Use:* Massage. *Internal Use:* Orally 3 to 5 drops in Solubol™ with water.

Intestinal System: Helps to relieve gas and constipation. *External Use:* Massage, reflexology. *Internal Use:* Orally 3 to 5 drops in Solubol™ with water.

Mind System: Stimulates motivation, direction, and the ability to change. *External Use:* Diffuse with citrus oils.

Muscular System: Muscle pain, stiffness, and fatigue. *External Use:* Massage, reflexology.

Nervous System: Stimulating. *External Use:* Massage, reflexology.

Reproductive System: Aphrodisiac, frigidity, impotence, toning to the uterus. *External Use:* Massage, reflexology.

Respiratory System: Helps to move mucous, expectorant. *External Use:* Diffuse, massage, reflexology.

Skeletal System: Rheumatic and arthritic pain, toothaches. *External Use:* Massage, reflexology.

Contraindication: Can irritate the skin.

*When diffusing, massaging and using reflexology, blend black pepper with other essential oils because of its tendency to irritate the skin. Use only 3% of black pepper.

Bois de Rose

(*Aniba parriflora*)
COUNTRY OF ORIGIN: Brazil
LAURACEAE FAMILY
It combines well with Lemon, Orange, Grapefruit, Sandalwood, Cedarwood, Pine and Spruce.

Major Chemical Constituents: linalool, α terpineol, geraniol.

The aroma is a very sweet floral with a hint of spice. Bois de Rose, or rosewood, is steam distilled. The part used in the extracting of this essence is the wood chips. This wild evergreen tree is found growing in the tropical Amazon. In Japan, chopsticks are made from this wood. The color is clear to a pale yellow.

Immune System: Antibacterial properties, helps with colds, flu, fevers and infections. It helps to get the system going. *External Use:* Bath, massage. *Internal Use:* Enema, suppositories.

Mind System: Helps to calm and steady emotions. *External Use:* Diffuse, massage, reflexology.

Nervous System: Frigidity, headaches, nausea associated with headaches, nervous tension, general stress; it is very calming. *External Use:* Diffuse, bath, massage, reflexology.

Reproductive System: Aphrodisiac, vaginitis, Candida Albicans. *Internal Use:* Suppositories, douche. *External Use:* Diffuse, massage, reflexology, bath.

Skin System: Toning effects, good for wrinkles and general skin care. Its balancing to the skin whether dry, oily or a combination of both. Used in perfumes and soaps. *External Use:* Facial, compress, bath.

Contraindication: Non-toxic, non-irritant.

Cedarwood

(Cedrus atlantica)
COUNTRY OF ORIGIN: Lebanon, Morocco
PINACEAE FAMILY
It combines well with Bois de Rose, Cypress and Bergamot.

Major Chemical Constituents: α himachalene, β himachalene, γ himachalene, d himachalene, γ atlantone Z, α atlantone E.

The aroma is warm, woody, sweet and slightly camphoric. Cedarwood is steam distilled. The part used in extracting this essence is the wood or sawdust. Cedrus Atlantica is a pine tree, believed to have originated in

Lebanon. It grows abundantly in the Atlantic Mountains. The color is yellowish to orange yellow to amber.

Circulatory System: Cellulite, fluid retention, circulation tonic, stimulating and toning encourages the flow of bile. *External Use:* Massage, reflexology.

Immune System: Antifungal. *External Use:* Massage, compress.

Lymphatic System: Cellulite, stimulating and toning, good for fluid retention. *External Use:* Massage.

Mind System: Irritation, agitation, anxiety, relaxant, nervous system, good for meditation, stabilizes. *External Use:* Diffuse, inhalation.

Reproductive System: Aphrodisiac, vaginal infections, gonorrhea. *External Use:* Massage. *Internal Use:* Suppositories, douche.

Respiratory System: Expectorant, catarrh, coughs, bronchitis. *External Use:* Compress, massage, ointment.

Skin System: Acne, cuts, wounds, greasy skin, scars, astringent, insect repellent, anti-fungal. *External Use:* Compress, clay pack, ointment.

Urinary System: Fluid retention, infection of the bladder. *External Use:* Massage, compress, reflexology.

Contraindications: Do not use during pregnancy or with high blood pressure.

Cistus

(Cistus landaniferus)
COUNTRY OF ORIGIN: Spain, Portugal
CISTATAE FAMILY
It combines well with Neroli, Lavender, Lemon, Tuberose, Cedar, Jasmine and Cypress.

Major Chemical Constituents: α pinene, bornyl acetate, trans-pino carveol, 2,2,6 trimethyl cyclohexanone

The aroma is warm, spicy, woody, tangy, soothing, and strong. Another name for Cistus is rock rose. The leaves of Cistus are steam distilled.

Circulatory System: Increases body temperature, increases circulation and helps with edema. *External Use:* Massage, reflexology.

Glandular System: Stimulates the glands to produce secretions. *External Use:* Ointment, diffuse, massage, reflexology.

Immune System: Stimulates white blood cells, whooping cough, measles and chicken pox. *External Use:* Massage, compress, reflexology.

Lymphatic System: Lymph congestion, swollen lymph glands. *External Use:* Massage, reflexology.

Mind System: Comforting, balancing, centering, inner emptiness, emotional coldness, frigidity and trauma. It aids in meditation, entering, focusing, visualizing, grounding, opening. Stimulating to the crown chakra. *External Use:* Diffuse, inhalation, massage, reflexology.

Muscular System: Reduces inflammation. *External Use:* Diffuse, inhalation, massage, compresses.

Reproductive System: Menstrual cramps. *External Use:* Massage, reflexology.

Skin System: Psoriasis, eczema, oily or dry skin, rough, callused, aging skin and acne. It's astringent and regenerative properties help to heal infected and ulcerated wounds. *External Use:* Bath, facial, ointment.

Urinary System: Inflammation of the bladder. *External Use:* Bath, massage, reflexology, acupressure, compress.

Contraindication: Do not use during pregnancy.

Cinnamon

(Cinnamomum zeylanicum)
COUNTRY OF ORIGIN: Sri Lanka, Africa, Indochina, Madagascar
LAURACEAE FAMILY

It combines well with: Clove, Orange, Lemon, Tangerine, Bergamot, Patchouli, Nutmeg, Coriander, Cardamon, Frankincense, Geranium, Ginger, Lemongrass, Peppermint, Rosemary, Bay, and Carrot.

Major Chemical Constituents: cinnamaldehyde, eugenol, cinnamyle acetate, linalool.

The aroma is spicy, stimulating, warm and sweet. Cinnamon is steam distilled. The part used in extracting this essence are the leaves and the bark. The color is a pale yellow to a brownish.

Circulatory System: Stimulating, helps with anemia, assists the heart in circulating the fluids. *Internal Use:* Orally 2 to 3 drops in Solubol™ with water twice daily.

Digestive System: Calming and warming, anti-spasmodic for stomach. *Internal Use:* Orally 2 to 3 drops in Solubol™ with water twice daily.

Immune System: Antibiotic for colds, flu, protection against contagious diseases. *Internal Use:* Orally 2 to 3 drops in Solubol™ with water three times daily.

Intestinal System: Helps with relief of gas and diaherra. Blends well with clove and lemon. *Internal Use:* Orally 2 to 3 drops in Solubol™ with water twice daily.

Mind System: Fear, emotional, coldness, tension, exhaustion, moodiness, heightens the physical senses, enhances creativity, pick me up for courage. Positive side of Cinnamon is its warming to the heart. *External Use:* Diffuse.

Reproductive System: Painful menstruation, aphrodisiac, impotence, stimulates contractions in childbirth. *Internal Use:* Orally 2 to 3 drops in Solubol ™ with water twice daily.

Skin System: Antiseptic for gingivitis. *External Use:* 3% cinnamon in aloe vera gel.

Contraindications: Do not diffuse alone, always blend with other essential oils. Do not use during pregnancy. Skin irritant. Do not use in bath or steam inhalation. Do not use on children under eight years of age. When using cinnamon only use 3% of it diluted in carrier oil. Do not use if you have hepatitis.

Clary Sage

(Salvia sclarea)

COUNTRY OF ORIGIN: U.S.S.R, Europe, Morocco, U.S.A.

LABIATAE FAMILY

It combines well with Bergamot, Lavender, Jasmine, Fennel, Neroli, Nutmeg, Petitgrain, Pine, Rose, Frnakincense, Vetiver, Juniper Berry, Mimosa, Sandalwood, Coriander, Cardamom, Roman Chamomile.

Major Chemical Constituents: linalool, linalyl acetate, germacrene D, geranyl acetate, sclareol.

The aroma is sweet, nutty, and herby. Clary sage is steam distilled. The parts used in the extracting of the essence are the flowering tops and foliage. It is clear to yellow to a light olive color.

Digestive System: Soothing to the stomach, poor digestion. *Internal Use:* Orally 2 to 3 drops Solubol.™ with water.

Immune System: Bacterial. *Internal Use:* Oally 2 to 3 drops Solubol™ with water.

Mind System: Depression, good for any kind of debilitation whether physical or mental. Great when in a weakened state. Fear, nervousness, hysteria, good for elderly when convalescing, postnatal depression. *External Use:* Massage, diffuse, reflexology, acupressure, inhalation.

Muscular System: Muscle pain and aches. *External Use:* Massage, reflexology, acupressure.

Nervous System: Sedative, calming, convulsions, migraines, headaches, hang-overs. *External Use:* Massage, bath, diffused, inhalation, reflexology.

Reproductive System: Toning for the uterus, aphrodisiac, premenstrual system, dysmenorrhea—painful and difficult menstruation, helps when not having a period (except during pregnancy). Frigidity, impotence, good for childbirth, menopause. *External Use:* Massage, bath, diffuser, reflexology.

Respiratory System: Throat infections, whooping cough. *External Use:* Gargle, massage, inhalation, diffuse.

Skin System: Scarring, ulcers, wrinkles, oily and dry skin, oily hair. *External Use:* Facial, massage, bath.

Contraindications: Do not use during pregnancy.

Clove

(Eugena caryophyllata)
COUNTRY OF ORIGIN: India, Madagascar
MYRTACEAE FAMILY
It combines well with Basil, Benzoin, Black Pepper, Cinnamon, Citronella, Grapefruit, Lemon, Orange, Peppermint, Clary Sage, Bergamot, Rosemary, Lavender, Geranium, Ginger, Palma Rosa, Sandalwood, Ylang Ylang, Ravensara, Nutmeg, and Bay.

Major Chemical Constituents: eugenol, eugenyle acetate, β caryophyllene.

The aroma is spicy, strong, penetrating, and warm. Clove is steam distilled. The part used for extracting the essence are the flower buds and flowery pedicels of the tree. The buds are called "cloves" and the pedicels are called "claws," because the top of the pedicels are crowned by a series of bracts in the shape of claws.

Circulatory System: Anemia, low blood pressure, stimulating to the circulation. *Internal Use:* Orally 2 to 3 drops in Solubol™ with water twice daily. *External Use:* Massage, reflexology.

Digestive System: Helps to expel gas from the stomach, and infections occurring in the stomach. *External Use:* Massage, relexology. *Internal Use:* Orally 2 to 3 drops in Solubol™ with water twice daily.

Immune System: Antiseptic for infectious diseases, stimulates the immune system when the body is deficient, combine with cinnamon for gastrointestinal illnesses, protection against contagious diseases, tuberculosis. Dental infections. *External Use:* Massage, reflexology. *Internal Use:* Orally 2 to 3 drops in Solubol™ with water twice daily.

Intestinal System: Infectious gastrointestinal illnesses, parasites, works well for the intestinal function when digesting heavy consumptions of red meat, cooked pork meat and cheese. *External Use:* Massage, reflexology. *Internal Use:* Orally 2 to 3 drops in Solubol™ with water twice daily.

Mind System: Stimulates positive thinking, strengthens memory, relieves depression, lethargy, fear, sadness, grief, despair, loneliness, nervous fatigue, stress, mental revitaliser, particularly for strongly emotional people. For anxiety, blend with Bay and Ravensara, especially when accepting full responsibility for one's life or in other words, cutting the umbilical cord. *External Use:* Diffuse, massage, reflexology, acupressure.

Nervous System: Nervous fatigue, energy deficiency, stimulates the chi, fights off drowsiness when combined with peppermint. *External Use:* Massage, reflexology, acupressure.

Reproductive System: Aphrodisiac, impotence, strengthens the uterus, aids in childbirth. It's a remarkable uterine tonic, it helps dilate the uterine muscles and thus prepares the mother for an easy birth physically, and also mentally, since it lessens anxiety about the delivery. *External Use:* Acupressure, massage, reflexology, compress. *Internal Use:* Orally 2 to 3 drops in Solubol™ with water twice daily.

Respiratory System: Antiseptic, and it stimulates the respiratory system. *External Use:* Massage, compresses, vaporizer.

Structural System: Muscular pain, toothache, general pain killer, dental infection. Not recommended for teething children. Antiseptic qualities-use as a mouthwash, gargle. *External Use:* Massage, compresses, vaporizer.

Urinary System: Urinary infections. *Internal Use:* Orally 2 to 3 drops in Solubol™ with water twice daily.

Contraindications: Do not use during pregnancy or on children under 8 years of age. Do not use if you have hepatitis.

Cypress

(Cupressus sempervirens)
COUNTRY OF ORIGIN: France
CYPRESSACEAE FAMILY
It combines well with Fennel, Bergamot, Clary Sage, Peppermint, Lemon, Lavender, Orange, Juniper, Pine, Sweet Thyme, Geranium, Vetiver, Niaouli, and Eucalyptus.

Major Chemical Constituents: α pinene, Δ 3 carene, cedrol, δ and γ cadinene.

The aroma is sweet-balsamic, refreshing odor, reminiscent of pine needles. Cypress is steam distilled. The parts used in the extracting of this essence are the leaves, needles and twigs. It can be clear to a pale yellow or pale olive green color.

Circulatory System: Varicose veins, increases circulation. *External Use:* Massage, Sitzbath, compress.

Digestive System: Internal bleeding. *Internal Use:* Orally 2 to 4 drops in Solubol™ with water three times daily.

Intestinal System: Diarrhea, hemorrhoids. *External Use:* Ointment. *Internal Use:* Suppositories, orally 2 to 4 drops in Solubol™ two or three times daily.

Immune System: Measles, chicken pox, and whooping cough. *Internal Use:* Orally 2 to 4 drops with Solubol™ and water three times daily.

Mind System: Absent minded, transitions, centering, focus, nervous breakdown, obsession with sex, uncontrollable sobbing, strength and comfort. *External Use:* Massage, bath, inhalation, diffuse.

Muscular System: Toning for weak muscles. *External Use:* Massage, bath, reflexology, compress.

Reproductive System: Menopause, ovarian cyst, dysmenorrhea. *External Use:* Massage, bath, reflexology, compress. *Internal Use:* Orally 2 to 4 drops in Solubol™ two or three times daily.

Respiratory System: Convulsive coughs, whooping coughs, expectorant. *External Use:* Inhalation. *Internal Use:* Orally 2 to 4 drops in Solubol™ two or three times daily.

Skin System: Deodorant of feet, astringent and toning properties, bleeding gums, oily skin and acne, scars, wounds. It is antiseptic for oily hair, dandruff. *External Use:* Compresses, facials, inhalations, shampoos, massage, clay packs.

Skeletal System: Arthritis, rheumatism. *External Use:* Massage, acupressure, reflexology, bath, compresses.

Urinary System: Diuretic. *Internal Use:* Orally 2 to 4 drops in Solubol™ two or three times daily.

Contraindications: None.

Dill

(Anethum graveolens)
COUNTRY OF ORIGIN: Mediterranean
UMBELLITERAE FAMILY
It combines well with Orange, Roman Chamomile, Lavender, Lemon, Tangerine, Rosemary, Basil, Sandalwood, Ravensara and Juniper.

Major Chemical Constituents: limonene, D carvone.

The aroma is fresh, peppery, sweet and spicy. Dill is steam distilled. The parts used in extracting of the essence are the seeds or the weed. It is an annual herb that makes an umbrella with its feathery leaves and yellowish flowers. The color ranges from clear to pale yellow.

Circulatory System: Stimulates circulation. *Internal Use:* Orally 2 to 3 drops in Solubol™ with water twice daily.

Digestive System: It is calming to the stomach, stimulates digestion, and works well with people who suffer with hiatial hernias. *External Use:* Massage on stomach blended with other oils such as citrus. *Internal Use:* Orally 3 to 4 drops in Solubol™ with water three times daily.

Intestinal System: Gas, colic, antispasmodic, colitis, irritable bowel syndrome, spastic colon, ileocecal valve problems. *External Use:* Massage, reflexology. *Internal Use:* Orally 3 to 4 drops in Solubol™ with water twice daily.

Mind System: Dill is helpful when we feel overwhelmed. In my personal opinion, when we are emotionally overwhelmed by worries and stresses, our centers of digestion and elimination tend not to work well. *External Use:* Diffusion, inhalation.

Reproductive System: Promotes milk flow in nursing mothers and stimulates the menses. *Internal Use:* Orally 2 to 3 drops in Solubol™ with water twice daily.

Respiratory System: Bronchitis. *Internal Use:* Orally 2 to 3 drops in Solubol™ with water twice daily, suppositories.

Urinary System: Dill works on the kidneys without irritation. *Internal Use:* Orally 2 to 3 drops in Solubol™ with water twice daily, suppositories.

Contraindications: Do not use during pregnancy. Do not use dill seed oil on children under 3; the whole weed needs to be used for children under 3.

Eucalyptus

(Eucalyptus globulus)
COUNTRY OF ORIGIN: Spain, Australia.
MYRTACEAE FAMILY
It combines well with Lemon, Lavender, Pine, Tea Tree, Thyme, Benzoin, Bay, Ravensara, Rosemary, Hyssop Peppermint, Chamomile and Cypress.

Major Chemical Constituents: 1, 8 cineol, limonene, trans-pino carveol, aromadendrene, globulol.

The aroma is fresh, balsamic, camphoric, pungent, dry, voluptuous, deep and tenacious. Eucalyptus is steam distilled. The parts used for extracting the essence are the leaves and branches. The color is clear to pale yellow.

Circulatory System: Angina, blood cleansing. *External Use:* Massage, ointments, compresses, diffusion, bath.

Digestive System: Gallstones, diabetes. *Internal Use:* Orally 3 to 4 drops in Solubol™ with water twice daily.

Glandular System: Hypoglycemia. *Internal Use:* Orally 3 to 4 drops in Solubol™ with water twice daily.

Immune System: Chicken pox, measles, scarlet fever, prevention of malaria, tuberculosis, candida, fever reducing, flu, sinus, colds, protection against contagious diseases. For cold sores and shingles blend with Bergamot. *External Use:* Compress, diffuse, reflexology, inhalation. *Internal Use:* Orally 2 to 3 drops in Solubol™ with water three times daily, suppositories.

Intestinal System: Intestinal parasites. *Internal Use:* Orally 2 to 3 drops in Solubol™ with water twice daily.

Mind System: Emotional balancer, concentration, centering, temper tantrums, cooling, mood swings, cluttered thoughts, argumentative, explosive nature. Very useful for recentering a scattered person who is the victim of respiratory spasms, symptoms for no longer being in balance with the world around in low amounts, it acts gently and patiently, and is a remarkable supplement to the other essential oils that help the Ego incarnate and as a result, assist in restoring the equilibrium. It helps us to reveal the best of ourselves. *External Use:* Diffuse, inhalation, massage, acupressure, bath, compress.

Nervous System: Herpes, shingles, and migraines. *External Use:* Massage, compress. *Internal Use:* orally 2 to 3 drops in Solubol™ with water twice daily.

Reproductive System: Relieving cramps. *External Use:* Compress, massage.

Respiratory System: Expectorant to the bottom of the respiratory function, air disinfectant, sinus infection, throat infection, croupy cough, bronchitis, tuberculosis. *External Use:* Ointments, compresses, diffusion, massage, inhalation, bath. *Internal Use:* Orally 2 to 3 drops in Solubol™ with water twice daily, suppositories.

Skeletal System: Fibrositis, muscular aches and pains, rheumatism. *External Use:* Compress, massage, reflexology.

Skin and Hair Systems: Ulcers on the skin, sunburn, diabetic sores and wounds, wound healing, shingles, herpes, chicken pox, measles, scarlet fever, dandruff, shampoos, deodorant, blemishes, acne and insect repellent. *External Use:* Ointments, compresses, diffusion, massage, inhalation, bath, shampoo.

Urinary System: Bladder infections. *Internal Use:* Orally 2 to 3 drops in Solubol™ with water twice daily.

Contraindications: Do not use on children under 2 years of age or asthmatics.

Fennel

(Foeniculum vulgare)
COUNTRY OF ORIGIN: France, Mediterranean, Asia, India
UMBELLIFERAE FAMILY
It combines well with Clary Sage, Rose, Lavender, Black Pepper, Cardamon, Ginger, Grapefruit, Lemon, Marjoram, Niaouli, Ravensara, Rosemary, Ylang Ylang and Sandalwood.

Major Chemical Constituents: fenchone, phellandrene, trans-anethole, anisaldehyde.

Fennel is steam distilled. The parts used for extracting the essence are the seeds. The color is clear to pale yellow. The aroma is licorice-like and deep.

Digestive System: Anorexia, increases appetite, colic, gas, nausea, painful and difficult digestion. Abdominal pains and cramps. *Internal Use:* Orally 2 to 3 drops in Solubol™ with water twice daily.

Glandular System: Hypoglycemia--balances blood sugar. *External Use:* Sniff directly from bottle. *Internal Use:* Orally 3 drops in Solubol™ with water tree times daily.

Immune System: Protection against influenza. *Internal Use:* Orally 2 to 3 drops in Solubol™ with water three times daily.

Intestinal System: Constipation. *Internal Use:* Orally 2 to 3 drops in Solubol™ with water twice dail, suppository.

Lymphatic System: Stimulates fluids helping with cellulite. *External Use:* Massage, reflexology.

Mind System: Unable to adjust, lack of creativity; Fennel helps to motivate our will forces and to carry on. *External Use:* Sniff directly from bottle.

Reproductive System: Stimulates menses, promotes milk in nursing mothers, and helps with engorgement of breast, menopause challenges, P.M.S. *Internal Use:* Orally 2 to 3 drops in Solubol™ with water twice daily.

Respiratory System: Expectorant, bronchitis. *Internal Use:* Orally 2 to 3 drops in Solubol™ with water three times daily.

Skin System: Bruises, dull oily complexion, pyorrhea. *External Use:* Compress, facial.

Urinary System: Edema-diuretic, kidney stones, and gout. *Internal Use:* Orally 2 to 3 drops in Solubol™ and water twice daily.

Contraindications: Do not use during pregnancy or epilepsy.

Frankincense

(Boswelia carterii)
COUNTRY OF ORIGIN: Somalia, Ethiopia
BURSERACEAE FAMILY
It combines well with: Myrrh, Basil, Cedarwood, Cypress, Elemi, Juniper Berry, Lavender, Neroli, Rose, Patchouli, Lemon, Sandalwood, Vetiver, Orange, Cinnamon and Coriander.

Major Chemical Constituents: α pinene, camphene, β pinene, sabinene, α terpinene, limonene,β phellandrene, p-cymene, octyle acetate, linalol, bornyl acetate, verbenone, viridflorol, incensol, incensyle acetate.

The aroma is warm, sweet, balsamic, spicy and incense-like. Frankincense is steam distilled. The part used in extracting the essence is the gum. The color is clear.

Immune System: Anti-infection, stimulating to the immune system, colds and flu. *External Use:* Massage, ointment, reflexology, acupressure, inhalation, diffuse.

Mind System: Meditation, to exalt the spirit, prayer, psychic abilities, cleansing of the mind, despair, apprehension, fear, grief. *External Use:* Diffuse, inhalation, reflexology, acupressure, massage.

Nervous System: Anxiety and nervous tension. *External Use:* Diffuse, inhalation, reflexology, massage, acupressure.

Reproductive System: Painful menstruation, P.M.S, breast inflammation, stress and nervous tension, uterine bleeding outside menstruation. *External Use:* Diffuse, inhalation, reflexology, massage, acupressure.

Respiratory System: Helps asthma, stimulates deep breathing, relaxing to the bronchial and chest, anti-catarrhal, expectorant(helps the lungs rid themselves of mucous) coughs, laryngitis. *External Use:* Diffuse, inhalation, reflexology, massage, acupressure. *Internal Use:* Suppositories.

Skin System: Analgesic, wounds, scars, wrinkles, acne, abscesses, toning. *External Use:* Facial, bath, massage, compresses, diffuse.

Urinary System: Infection of the bladder. *External Use:* Bath, compress, massage.

Contraindications: Avoid during first trimester of pregnancy.

Geranium

(Pelargonium asperum)
COUNTRY OF ORIGIN: Egypt, China, Madagascar
GERANIACENE FAMILY
It combines well with Juniper, Rose, Neroli, Clove, Patchouli, Lavender, Bergamot, Rosemary, Jasmine, Cypress and Sandalwood.

Major Chemical Constituents: cis-rose oxyde, trans-rose oxyde, citronellol, geraniol

The aroma is green, rosy, sweet and flowery. Geranium is steam distilled. The parts used in the extracting the essence are the stalks, leaves and flowers.

Circulatory System: Stimulates the heart, varicose veins, it stops bleeding when cut, poor circulation-cold hands and feet, and edema. *External Use:* Massage, bath, diffuse.

Digestive System: Helps diabetes, stimulates digestion, tonic for the liver and gallbladder. *External Use:* Compress, massage. *Internal Use:* Orally 2 to 3 drops in Solubol™ with water twice daily.

Glandular System: Balancing to the adrenals. *Internal Use:* Orally 3 to 5 drops in Solubol™ with water twice daily.

Immune System: Antibacterial, antibiotic, antiseptic, antifungal, helps with cold sores, herpes, shingles, and cell regeneration. *External Use:* Massage, bath, diffuse, inhalation, compress. *Internal Use:* Orally 2 to 4 drops in Solubol™ with water three times daily.

Intestinal System: Relieves hemorrhoids, intestinal catarrh and diarrhea. *Internal Use:* Orally, 2 to 3 drops in Solubol™ with water, suppositories, salve and ointment.

Mind System: It is great for therapy work (inner child). Anxiety, depression, consoling, rigidity, instability, moodiness, insecurity, low self esteem, overly sensitive, tension, stress, irritability, nervousness, acute fear, worry, discontent, and heartache. It creates harmony and good humor between the sexes and irons out irrationality and discontentment. *External Use:* Diffuse, inhalation, massage, compress, bath, reflexology, acupressure.

Nervous System: Good for depression, facial neuralgia, shingles, nervous fatigue, anxiety. *External Use:* Massage, bath, diffuse.

Reproductive System: Helps with menopause, endometrosis, P.M.S, infertility, vaginal bleeding, hormonal disturbances, painful periods, breast and uterine cancer, postpartum blues and impotence. During pregnancy, it is good for poor circulation, edema, stress, anxiety, breast engorgement and conditions of uterus. *Internal Use:* Orally 3 to 5 drops in Solubol™ with water twice daily, suppositories. *External Use:* Massage, compresses, reflexology.

Respiratory System: Sore throats. *Internal Use:* Gargle.

Skin and Hair Systems: It balances oily skin, dry and oily skin with dry patches; it heals wounds, frostbite, bruises, stress marks, scars, skin ulcers, sores on tongue, and mucous membranes. It is used as an insect repellent for mosquitoes and by the perfumery industry. *External Use:* Bath, massage, facials, diffuse, ointment, perfume.

Contraindications: None.

Ginger

(Zingiber officinale)
COUNTRY OF ORIGIN: Tropical India
ZINGIBERACEASE FAMILY
It combines well with Nutmeg, Clove, Bois de Rose, Coriander, Cedarwood, Lemon, Orange, Neroli, Juniper, Rosemary, Oregano, Roman Chamomile and Peppermint.

Major Chemical Constituents: zingiberene, geranyl acetate, β bis-abolene, α curcumene

The aroma is warm, spicy, fresh and sweet. Ginger is steam distilled. The part used in the extracting of this essence is the root. Ginger is native to the tropical coastal regions of India. The color is yellow.

Digestive System: Warms the stomach, stimulating digestion, good for motion sickness on boats and in cars, loss of appetite, nausea, vomiting, anorexia. *External Use:* Massage, bath, compress. *Internal Use:* Orally 2 to 3 drops in Solubol™ with water twice daily.

Immune System: Protection against contagious disease, colds, flu, chills. *Internal Use:* Orally 2 to 3 drops in Solubol™ with water twice daily.

Intestinal System: Helps to relieve gas and spasms, as well as diarrhea. *External Use:* Massage, bath, compress. *Internal Use:* Orally 2 to 3 drops in Solubol™ with water twice daily.

Mind System: Just like its aroma, ginger helps us to take action. It's warm and revitalizing, helps stimulate the memory. *External Use:* Massage, bath, compress.

Muscular System: For leg cramps and pain. *External Use:* Massage, compress, bath, a few drops in tub for only 15 minutes, or use in reflexology and acupressure. *Internal Use:* Orally 2 to 3 drops in Solubol™ with water twice daily.

Reproductive System: Used to help menstrual cramps and impotence. *External Use:* Massage, compress. *Internal Use:* Orally 2 to 3 drops in Solubol™ with water twice daily.

Respiratory System: A moist cough. *External Use:* Compresses, inhalation, bath.

Skeletal System: Rheumatism, arthritic pain. *External Use:* Massage.
Contraindications: May irritate sensitive skin.

Grapefruit

(Citrus paradisi)
COUNTRY OF ORIGIN: Asia, U.S.A, Israel, Brazil.

RUTACEAE FAMILY

It combines well with Ginger, Juniper, Cypress, Clary Sage, Clove, Palmarosa, Ylang Ylang, Mandarin, Cardamom, Patchouli, Thyme, Neroli, Lavender, Geranium, Rosemary, Peppermint, Eucalyptus, Fennel, Black Pepper, Frankincense and Nutmeg.

Major Chemical constituents: limonene, γ terpinene, nootkatone, cadinene, neral, citronell, Δ cadinene geranial.

The aroma is warm, sweet, fresh and sparkling citrus. The rind of grapefruit is cold pressed. The color is yellowish to a greenish yellow.

Circulatory System: Stimulating to the circulation. *External Use:* Massage.

Digestive System: Helps aid in digestion. *Internal Use:* Orally 2 to 3 drops in Solubol™ with water twice daily.

Immune System: Flu, colds, chills, anti-infectious, disinfectant, anti-septic. *External Use:* Massage, reflexology, bath, diffuse. *Internal Use:* Orally 2 to 3 drops in Solubol™ with water twice daily.

Intestinal System: Cleansing. *Internal Use:* Orally 2 to 3 drops in Solubol™ with water twice daily.

Lymphatic System: Toning, restorative to the lymph glands, detoxify-ing, cellulite, obesity. *External Use:* Massage, reflexology, bath.

Mind System: Confidence, clarity, to relieve depression. *External Use:* Massage, diffuse, inhalation.

Muscular System: Aches and pains (exercise preparation). *External Use:* Massage, bath.

Nervous System: Headaches, nervous exhaustion, depression, stress due to pressure. *External Use:* Massage, diffuse, reflexology.

Skeletal System: Joint pain. *External Use:* Massage, bath, reflexology.

Skin System: Congested and oily skin, acne, tones the skin, antiseptic for the skin. *External Use:* Facials, massage, diffuse.

Urinary System: Fluid retention. *Internal Use:* Orally 2 to 3 drops in Solubol™ with water twice daily.

Contraindication: Phototoxic.

Helichrysum

(Helichrysum italicum g. don)
COUNTRY OF ORIGIN: Mediterranean
COMPOSITAE FAMILY
It combines well with Orange, Lemon, Chamomile, Geranium, Rose, Lavender, Neroli, Clove and Clary Sage.

Major Chemical Constituents: neryle acetate, nerol, diomes

The aroma is sweetly rich and overwhelming, honey-like. Helichrysum is steam distilled. The parts used in the extracting process are the flowers. It can sometimes be called immortelle or everlast. The color is a pale yellow.

Circulatory System: Increase circulation, helps with bruising and hemorrhage. *Internal Use:* Hemorrhage oil, orally 2 to 3 drops in Solubol™ with water twice daily. *External Use:* Massage, compress, bath, ointment.

Digestive System: Spleen and liver congestion. *Internal Use:* Orally 2 to 3 drops in Solubol™ with water twice daily.

Immune System: Antimicrobial, good for colds, flu, fevers, bacterial infections. *External Use:* Diffuse, massage, compress, reflexology. *Internal Use:* Orally 2 to 3 drops in Solubol™ with water twice daily.

Mind System: Depression, stress, tension, tiredness. It is warming and brings forth harmony to the emotions. *External Use:* Diffuse, massage, bath, compress.

Muscular System: Anti-inflammatory, helps relieve muscle pain and tension, sprains and strains. *External Use:* Massage, reflexology, acupressure, bath, compress.

Nervous System: Depression, stress, nervous fatigue, sharp, stabbing pain along the nerves. *External Use:* Massage, reflexology, acupressure, bath, compress.

Respiratory System: Relieves coughs, asthma, bronchitis, whooping cough. *Internal Use:* Orally 2 to 3 drops in Solubol™ with water twice daily.

Skeletal System: Helps rheumatism with its anti-inflammatory properties. *External Use:* Massage, reflexology, acupressure, bath, compress.

Skin System: Scars, bruises. *External Use:* Ointment, compress, bath, massage.

Contraindications: None.

Hyssop

(Hyssops officinalis)
COUNTRY OF ORIGIN: Mediterranean
LABIATAE FAMILY
It combines well with Bay, Lemon, Lavender, Geranium, Clary Sage, Orange, Rosemary and Grapefruit.

Major Chemical Constituents: iso pinocamphone, pinocamphone δ germacrene D.

The aroma is sweet, camphoric, with warm spicy undertones. Hyssop is steam distilled. The part used in the extracting of this essence is the plant. It is clear to a pale yellowy green.

Circulatory System: Low blood pressure. *Internal Use:* Orally 2 to 3 drops in Solubol™ with water three times daily.

Digestive System: Loss of appetite, slow digestion, distention of stomach, stomach pain due to nerves. *Internal Use:* Orally 2 to 3 drops in Solubol™ with water three times daily.

Intestinal System: Intestinal parasites. *Internal Use:* Orally 2 to 3 drops in Solubol™ with water three times daily.

Immune System: Bronchitis, protection against influenza, tuberculosis. *Internal Use:* Orally 2 to 4 drops three times daily in Solubol™ with water three times daily.

Reproductive System: Helps with heavy vaginal discharge and scanty periods. *Internal Use:* Orally 2 to 3 drops in Solubol™ with water three times daily.

Respiratory System: Asthma, hay fever, chronic bronchitis, cough, influenza, and tuberculosis. *Internal Use:* Orally 2 to 3 drops in Solubol™ with water three times daily.

Skeletal System: For rheumatism. *Internal Use:* Orally 2 to 3 drops in Solubol™ with water three times daily.

Skin System: Works on scars, wounds, bruises, eczema. *External Use:* Compresses, massage, reflexology, ointments.

Contraindications: Do not use during pregnancy. High doses are toxic and cause epileptic seizures.

Jasmine

(Jasminium grandiflorum)
COUNTRY OF ORIGIN: Iran
OLEACEAE FAMILY

It combines well with Rose, Ylang Ylang, Sandalwood, Bergamot, Pettigrain, Orange, Lemon, Palmarosa, Geranium and Rosewood.

Major Chemical Constituents: benzyl acetate, benzyl benzonate, linalool, butyl acetate, isophytol.

The aroma is intensely heavy with warm, rich, floral, and exotic tea like undertones. Jasmine is a solvent extract. The color is orange to a brown color.

Mind System: Postpartum blues, frigidity, anger, worry. Alleviates fear, sadness, low self esteem. It is inspiring, encouraging, and warming to the emotions. *External Use:* Inhalation, massage, reflexology, acupressure.

Reproductive System: The toning effects of Jasmine have widely been used for female and male reproductive challenges: In women it helps with the relief of menstrual cramps and pain. It has also been beneficial in childbirth, helping to make the contractions harder, making expulsion easier, and warms the womb to help facilitate birth. Emotionally it helps with postpartum blues and frigidity. For men its toning effects help with enlargement of the prostate. Historically, it has been used for its aphrodisiac qualities, relaxing both partners, helping them to enjoy themselves. *External Use:* Massage, bath, reflexology, acupressure, ointment.

Respiratory System: Coughs, expectorant, laryngitis. *External Use:* Inhalation, massage, bath, ointment.

Skin System: For dry, sensitive, mature skin, stress related skin disorders, acne. *External Use:* Facial, compress, ointment.

Contraindications: Do not use during pregnancy, only during childbirth.

*Best used as an ointment or in massage.

Juniper

(Juniperus communis)
COUNTRY OF ORIGIN: France.
CUPRESSACEAE FAMILY
It combines well with: Eucalyptus, Mandarin, Cypress, Clary Sage, Benzoin, Bergamot, Frankincense, Sandalwood, Thyme, Rosemary and Geranium.

Major Chemical Constituents: *Berries:* α pinene, sabinene, myrcene, germacrene D, δ cadinene, γ cadinene. *Branches:* α pinene, sabinene, myrcene, terpinene 4 ol, thujopsene.

The aroma is fresh, sweet, warm, and balsamic. Juniper is steam distilled. The parts used in the extracting of this essence are the juniper berries and branches. The color is clear to pale yellow.

Circulatory System: Increases circulation, arteriosclerosis. *Internal Use:* Orally 2 to 3 drops in Solubol™ with water twice daily. *External Use:* Massage, bath, compress, reflexology, acupressure.

Digestive System: Stimulates the pancreas, helps with loss of appetite, cirrhosis, and indigestion. *Internal Use:* Orally 2 to 3 drops in Solubol™ with water twice daily. *External Use:* Massage, bath, compress, reflexology, acupressure.

Intestinal System: Intestinal ferment. *Internal Use:* Orally 2 to 3 drops in Solubol™ with water twice daily. *External Use:* Massage, bath, compress.

Immune System: Antiseptic, protects against contagious disease, gonorrhea. *Internal Use:* Orally 2 to 3 drops in Solubol™ with water.

Lymphatic System: Stimulates the fluids in the body, helping the body to rid itself of toxins, cellulite and gout. *External Use:* Massage, compress, reflexology, acupressure.

Mind System: Purifies and cleanses the mind of confusion and depletion from being with others. Helps enhance and support meditation and prayer. *External Use:* Diffuse, massage, reflexology, bath, acupressure, compress.

Nervous System: Anxiety, nervous tension. *External Use:* massage, bath, acupressure, reflexology, compress, diffuse.

Reproductive System: Stimulates menstruation, painful periods, aphrodisiac, gonorrhea. *Internal Use:* Orally 2 to 3 drops in Solubol™ with water twice daily. *External Use:* Massage, compress, reflexology, bath, acupressure.

Skeletal System: Rheumatism, arthritis. *External Use:* Bath, compress, reflexology, acupressure.

Skin System: Scars, wounds, weeping, eczema, acne, dandruff. *External Use:* Massage, bath, compress, salve, shampoo.

Urinary System: Infection of bladder. *Internal Use:* Orally 2 to 3 drops in Solubol™ with water twice daily.

Contraindications: Do not use during pregnancy or in kidney disease.

Lavender

(Lavandula angustifolia)
COUNTRY OF ORIGIN: France
LAMIACEASE LABIATAE FAMILY
It combines well with almost all other essential oils.

Major Chemical Constituents: linalyl acetate, linalool, cis and trans β ocimene, lavandulyle acetate, terpinene 4 ol.

The aroma is mellow, peaceful, but can be overwhelming. Lavender is steam distilled. The parts used in extracting the essence are the flowers, stalks and leaves. It is clear to a pale yellow.

Circulatory System: Palpitations, high blood pressure, restores and tones the heart. *External Use:* Massage, bath, diffuse.

Digestive System: Helps to expel gas from the stomach and aids in healing ulcers. *External Use:* Massage, compress.

Immune System: Antimicrobial, infections, fevers, antibiotic, sore throat, earache, antiseptic, whooping cough, protection against influenza, pulmonary tuberculosis and terminally ill, gargle. *External Use:* Massage, reflexology, acupressure, compresses, inhalation.

Intestinal System: Intestinal parasites, gas. *External Use:* Massage, reflexology, compress, acupressure.

Mind System: Irritability, stress, tension, mental exhaustion, panic, shock, anxiety, hysteria, apprehension, fears, nightmares, insecurity, lost inner child, restlessness, moodiness, distracted, addictions, obsessive behavior, trauma, conflict, emotional violence, agitation, jitters, depression, nervousness, worry, and burnout. *External Use:* Diffuse, massage, bath, inhalation.

Nervous System: Relaxing, calming, anti-convulsant, headaches from stress or tension, anxiety, convalescence, migraines, links the two sides of the brain, sedative, vertigo, epilepsy, insomnia, and high blood pressure. *External Use:* Diffuse, massage, bath.

Reproductive System: Painful periods, P.M.S, vaginitis, frigidity, scanty periods, gonorrhea, vaginitis. *Internal Use:* Suppositories, and douche. *External Use:* Massage, reflexology, compress, acupressure, bath.

Respiratory System: Coughs, asthma, earache, decongestant, influenza, tuberculosis, pulmonary, whooping cough. *External Use:* Diffuse, massage, bath.

Skeletal System: Inflammatory conditions, arthritis, rheumatism, osteoporosis, sprains. *External Use:* Massage, bath, compress, diffuse.

Skin and Hair Systems: Opens pores, stretch marks, sunburn, dry skin, scars, gout, antiseptic, disinfectant, athletes foot, eczema, psoriasis, insect bites, acne, abscesses, boils, anti-aging, wounds, ulcers, burn. It is used in shampoos, soaps, and all kinds of cosmetics. *External*

Use: Massage, bath, facials, diffuse.

Urinary System: Kidneys and fluid retention. *External Use:* Bath, massage, reflexology.

Contraindications: None.

Lemon

(Citrus limonuom)

COUNTRY OF ORIGIN: East India, U.S.A.

RUTACEAE FAMILY

It combines well with Cardamon, Lavender, Linden, Chamomile, Eucalyptus, Fennel, Ginger, Juniper, Neroli, Petigrain, Frankincense, Clove, Thyme, Geranium, Tea Tree, Sandalwood, Peppermint and Ylang Ylang.

Major Chemical Constituents: limonene, neral, geranial, neryl, δ geranyle, α terpinene.

The aroma is fresh and sharp. It synergizes well in blends. The lemon rind is cold pressed or distilled. The part used in the extracting is the rind. The color is a sunny golden yellow.

Circulatory System: Anemia, water retention, hardening of the arteries, varicose veins ,high blood pressure. *Internal Use:* Orally 2 to 3 drops in Solubol™ with water twice daily.

Digestive System: Gallbladder congestion such as gallstones, liver tonic, neutralizes acid, jaundice, vomiting, calming to the stomach, loss of appetite, stomach odors. *Internal Use:* Orally 2 to 3 drops in Solubol™ with water twice daily.

Immune System: Antiseptic, immune stimulant, it stimulates the white corpuscles, anti-viral, infectious diseases, colds, flu, sore throats, influenza when accompanied by a high fever, preventive of influenza, herpes, tuberculosis, pulmonary, malaria, syphilis, gonorrhea. *External Use:* Bath, massage, diffuse, inhalation. *Internal Use:* Orally 2 to 3 drops in Solubol™ with water twice daily, gargles.

Intestinal System: Intestinal parasites, infection of the intestines.

Internal Use: Orally 2 to 3 drops in Solubol™ with water twice daily.
External Use: Massage, reflexology, acupressure.

Lymphatic System: Cellulite, obesity. *External Use:* Massage, bath. *Internal Use:* Orally 2 to 3 drops in Solubol™ with water twice daily.

Mind System: It relaxes yet stimulates. Humorless, indecisive, bitter, bad attitude, apathetic, distrust, mental blocks, stress, mental fatigue, turmoil, irrationality, fear. It brings out joy, lively conscious awareness, direction, memory, versatility, and purifying. *External Use:* Massage, diffuse, inhalation.

Nervous System: Headaches, as well as migraine headaches, hypertension. *External Use:* Massage, diffuse, bath, reflexology.

Reproductive System: During pregnancy, it helps to tone the circulation, and reduce tissue congestion, also stimulates the immune system, improving the user's resistance to syphilis and gonorrhea. *External Use:* Massage, ointment, compress, reflexology. *Internal Use:* Orally 2 to 3 drops in Solubol™ with water twice daily.

Respiratory System: Asthma, bronchitis, pneumonia, sore throats. *External Use:* Compress, massage, reflexology, diffuse, inhalation. *Internal Use:* Orally 2 to 3 drops in Solubol™ with water twice daily, gargle.

Skeletal System: Rheumatism, arthritis, gout. *External Use:* Compress, massage, reflexology.

Skin and Hair Systems: For oily skin, wrinkles, cuts, wounds, scars, brittle nails, tender feet, helps to stop bleeding, mouth ulcers, gum tonic, freckles, corns, warts, for nose bleeds soak a small pad of cotton or wool and insert into nostril, insect bites, brittle nails. *External Use:* Facials, massage, compresses.

Urinary System: Water retention and also purifies the water we drink. Helps to dissolve kidney stones. *Internal Use:* Orally 2 to 3 drops in Solubol™ with water twice daily.

Contraindications: Although safe throughout pregnancy, it is phototoxic and may cause skin irritation.

Lemongrass

(Cymbopogori citratus)
COUNTRY OF ORIGIN: India, Madagascar.
GRAMINACEAE FAMILY
It combines well with Myrrh, Clove, Rosemary, Palma Rosa, Ginger, Patchouli, Eucalyptus, Geranium and Lavender.

Major Chemical Constituents: neral, geranial.

The aroma is fresh, citrus-like and reminiscent of herbal tea. Lemongrass is steam distilled. The part used in extracting is the tall grass. The color is yellow to amber color.

Circulatory System: Stimulates circulation. *Internal Use:* Orally 2 to 3 drops in Solubol™ with water twice daily.

Digestive System: Calming and stimulates digestion. *Internal Use:* Orally 2 to 3 drops in Solubol™ with water three times daily.

Immune System: Antibacterial for infections, antiviral, antifungal, fevers. *Internal Use:* Orally 2 to 3 drops in Solubol™ with water, gargles.

Intestinal System: Gas, parasites, and colic. *Internal Use:* Orally 2 to 3 drops in Solubol™ with water twice daily.

Muscular System: Relieves pain and tones the muscles, anti-inflammatory. *External Use:* Compress, massage, reflexology.

Nervous System: Helps with headaches because of it's sedative properties. *Internal Use:* Orally 2 to 3 drops in Solubol™ with water twice daily.

Reproductive System: Increases milk production. *Internal Use:* Orally 1 to 2 drops in Solubol™ with water twice daily.

Skin System: Insect repellent, acne, athlete's foot, lice, cold sores, shingles, scabies, and open pores. *External Use:* Deodorant, facials, massage, compresses.

Contraindications: Possible skin irritation.

Myrrh

(Commiphora myrrha)
COUNTRY OF ORIGIN: North East Africa.
BURSERACEAE FAMILY
It combines well with Cypress, Frankincense, Juniper Berry, Mandarin, Petitgrain, Cedarwood, Coriander Geranium, Lemongrass, Palmarosa and Patchouli.

Major Chemical Constituents: β elemene curzerene, heerabolene.

The aroma is deep, warm, spicy and slightly sweet. Myrrh is steam distilled from the resin of the tree. Its color is pale yellow to a pale orange.

Digestive System: It is stimulating to the whole digestive tract and encourages good digestion. *External Use:* Massage, reflexology, bath, inhalation.

Glandular System: Helps to balance the thyroid. *External Use:* Massage, reflexology.

Immune System: Anti-infectious. *External Use:* Bath, inhalation, massage, reflexology, and ointments. *Internal Use:* Suppositories.

Intestinal System: Crohn's disease, diarrhea, hemorrhoids. *External Use:* Massage, suppositories, enema, or colonic.

Mind System: Aids in prayer, meditation, supportive and strengthening. *External Use:* Reflexology, inhalation, bath, massage.

Reproductive System: Vaginitis, candida albicans infection, stimulates menstruation, uterine hemorrhage. *Internal Use:* Douche, suppositories.

Respiratory System: The anti-microbial and expectorant properties are helpful for bronchitis, colds, sore throats, chest infections. *External Use:* Massage, bath, inhalation, reflexology. *Internal Use:* Suppositories.

Skeletal System: The anti-inflammatory properties help with arthritic conditions. *External Use:* Massage, reflexology, acupressure.

Skin System: It's antiseptic properties help to heal wounds and scars. The astringent properties work well on receding gums, and mouth ulcers. Myrrh is also valued for its antiseptic properties. It works on athlete's foot, ringworm, jock itch, and thrush. It is also beneficial to dry, chapped, cracking skin and weeping eczema. *External Use:* Ointments, massage, facials, bath. *Internal Use:* Gargle, toothpaste.

Contraindications: Do not use during pregnancy.

Neroli

(Citrus aurantium)
COUNTRY OF ORIGIN: Tunisia, New Guinea.
.RUTACEAE FAMILY
It combines well with Geranium, Rose, Bergamot, Jasmine, Roman Chamomile, Lavender, Mandarin, Orange, Nerol, Geranium, Ylang Ylang, Ginger, Palmarosa, Sandalwood and Juniper.

Major Chemical Constituents: linalool, linalyle acetate, trans-trans-nerolidol, trans-trans-farnesol.

The aroma is inspiringly sweet and floral. Neroli is steam distilled. The parts used for extracting the essence are the flowers. Besides rose, neroli is the other oil, that can be used in all aspects of aromatherapy. The color is pale yellow.

Digestive System: Painful and difficult digestion due to nerves, colic. *Internal Use:* Orally 1 to 3 drops in Solubol™ with water twice daily.
Immune System: Candida Albicans. *Internal Use:* Orally 2 to 3 drops in Solubol™ with water three times daily, suppositories.
Intestinal System: balances the intestinal flora, chronic diarrhea, anti-infectious. *Internal Use:* Orally 1 to 3 drops in Solubol™ with water twice daily, suppositories.
Mind System: Shock, fear, depression, tension. It calms and stabilizes. It allows one to be at peace and feel light and loving. *External Use:* Diffuse, inhalation, massage, bath, reflexology.
Nervous System: Calming, soothing, insomnia, fear, shock, convalescence, depression, tension. *External Use:* Diffuse, inhalation, massage, bath, reflexology.
Reproductive System: P.M.S., vaginitis, Candida Albicans. *External Use:*

Massage, reflexology, bath. *Internal Use:* Suppositories, douche.
Skin System: Perfume, scars, stretchmarks. *External Use:* Facial, diffuse, steam inhalation, massage, bath.

Contraindications: None

Niaouli MQV

(Melaleuca viridiflora)
COUNTRY OF ORIGIN: New Caledonia, Madagascar.
MYRTACEAE FAMILY
It combines well with Lemon, Tea Tree, Ravensara, Rosemary, Peppermint, Roman Chamomile, Lavender and Geranium.

Major Chemical Constituents: 1, 8 cineol, α terpinolene, virdifloral.

The aroma is sweet, fresh, camphoric. Niaouli is steam distilled. The parts used for extracting the essence are the leaves. The color is a pale yellow to a greenish color.

Immune System: *Candida albicans,* strep throat, antibacterial, antiviral. It protects against influenza, tuberculosis, whooping cough. *External Use:* Massage, reflexology, compress, bath. *Internal Use:* Orally 5 to 6 drops in Solubol™ with water three times daily, gargle.
Intestinal System: Intestinal parasites. *Internal Use:* Orally use 2 to 3 drops in Solubol™ and water twice daily.
Reproductive System: Antiseptic for infection due to childbirth, cancer of vagina, dysplasia and cancer of breast. *External Use:* Massage. *Internal Use:* Orally use 2 to 3 drops in Solubol™ with water, suppositories.
Respiratory System: Antiseptic for the bronchioles, anti-catarrhal, chronic bronchitis, strep throat, whooping cough, asthma, pneumonia, pulmonary tuberculosis, sinus, nasal catarrhal, head cold. *External Use:* Compresses, inhalations, diffuse, bath, massage. *Internal Use:* Orally use 2 to 3 drops in Solubol™ with water, gargle.
Skeletal System: Analgesic for rheumatism. *Internal Use:* Orally use 2 to 3 drops in Solubol™ with water twice daily.

Skin System: Antiseptic for wounds, helps to heal scars, ulcers, burns, fistula. *External Use:* Ointment, fistula-bath, lotion, compresses.

Urinary System: Infection of the bladder and urethra. *Internal Use:* Orally use 2 to 3 drops of Solubol™ and water three times daily.

Contraindications: None.

Nutmeg

(Myristica Fragrans)
COUNTRY OF ORIGIN: Indonesia
MYRISTISACEAE FAMILY
It combines well with Clove, Roman Chamomile, Clary Sage, Rose and Ylang Ylang.

Major Chemical Constituents: α and β pinere, sabinene, myristicine, safrole.

The aroma is light, fresh, warm, spicy, sweet and somewhat woody. Nutmeg is steam distilled. The parts used are freshly dried nutmegs. The color is clear to a pale yellow.

Circulatory System: Stimulate circulation to the brain. *Internal Use:* Orally 2 to 3 drops in Solubol™ with water twice daily.

Digestive System: Calms and helps the stomach to digest food like mutton and starchy foods, dissolves gallstones, and increases appetite. *External Use:* Massage, reflexology. *Internal Use:* Orally 2 to 3 drops in Solubol™ with water twice daily.

Intestinal System: Intestinal infections, chronic diarrhea, gas. *Internal Use:* Orally 2 to 3 drops in Solubol™ with water twice daily.

Muscular System: Analgesic properties help alleviate muscle pain and tenseness. *External Use:* Massage, reflexology, acupressure.

Reproductive System: Stimulates menses. *External Use:* Massage, reflexology *Internal Use:* Orally 2 to 3 drops in Solubol™ with water twice daily..

Skin System: Helps to alleviate toothache pain. *External Use:* Massage gum area.

Contraindications: Do not use during pregnancy, only delivery.

Orange

(Citrus sinensis)
COUNTRY OF ORIGIN: Far East in Himalayas, Brazil, U.S.A.
RUTACEA FAMILY
It combines well with Black Pepper, Ylang Ylang, Sandalwood, Cinnamon, Clove, Patchouli, Geranium, Juniper, Rose, Frankincense and Jasmine.

Major Chemical Constituents: limonene.

The aroma is fresh, sweet and fruity. Orange is cold compressed. It is a coriander of grapefruit, lemon and vetiver. These trees originated in the Far East between the Himalayas and Southwest China. The color is yellow to orange.

Circulatory System: Calming to the heart. *External Use:* Massage, reflexology, acupressure.
Digestive System: Overindulgence, helps the stomach to digest better. *Internal Use:* Orally 2 to 3 drops in Solubol™ with water three to four times daily.
Immune System: Antibiotic properties, great for winter colds, antiseptic. *External Use:* Compress. *Internal Use:* Orally 2 to 3 drops in Solubol™ with water three to four times daily.
Intestinal System: Constipation, diarrhea. *Internal Use:* Orally 2 to 3 drops in Solubol™ with water three to four times daily.
Lymphatic System: Stimulates the fluids in the body. Cellulite, helps the body to rid itself of toxins. *External Use:* Massage, reflexology, acupressure.
Nervous System: Anxiety, insomnia. *External Use:* Inhalation, diffuse, massage, reflexology.
Mind System: Depression, sadness, burnout. Orange warms the heart and energizes. *External Use:* Diffuse, inhalation, massage, reflexology.
Skin System: Toning effects help with gums and mouth ulcers, acne. *Internal Use:* Gargle. *External Use:* Acne-clay mask, compress.

Urinary System: Diuretic, kidney stones. *Internal Use:* Orally 1 drop in Solubol™ with water three to four times daily.

Contraindications: Phototoxic.

Patchouli

(Pogostemon patchouli)
COUNTRY OF ORIGIN: Philippines, Indonesia
LABIATAE FAMILY
It combines well with Bergamot, Black Pepper, Geranium, Clove, Lavender, Ginger, Ylang Ylang, Lemongrass, Vetiver, Orange, Sandalwood, Neroli, Clary Sage and Mandarin.

Major Chemical Constituents: patchoulol, α guaiene, α and β patchoulene, seychellene.

The aroma is hot, earthy, musky and pungent. Patchouli is steam distilled. The parts used for extracting the essence are the dried leaves. The color is dark orange to brown.

Digestive System: Calming to the stomach, good to stop vomiting. *External Use:* Massage, bath compress, reflexology.

Immune System: Antifungal, antibacterial, antiviral. *External Use:* Bath, compress, massage, reflexology.

Lymphatic System: Obesity. *External Use:* Massage, reflexology, bath.

Mind System: Antidepressant, exhaustion, stress, anxiety, mood swings, indecision. *External Use:* Reflexology, spritzers, massage, acupressure, bath.

Nervous System: Frigidity, anxiety, nervousness, exhaustion, stress, stimulating to the nervous system. *External Use:* Bath, massage, compress, reflexology, acupressure.

Reproductive System: Aphrodisiac, frigidity. *External Use:* Massage, reflexology, acupressure.

Skeletal System: Anti-inflammatory. *External Use:* Compress, bath, reflexology.

Skin and Hair Systems: Acne, boils, wounds, scarring, cracked and chapped skin, eczema, sores, open pores, insect bites, ringworm, dandruff and anti-fungal infections, such as athlete's foot. Also used to regenerate cells, and in shampoo and perfumes. *External Use:* Bath, compress, spritz, ointment.

Urinary System: Diuretic, fluid retention. *External Use:* Massage, reflexology, acupressure, compress, bath.

Contraindications: Can be irritating.

Peppermint

(Mentha piperita)
COUNTRY OF ORIGIN: Oregon, U.S.A.
LABIATAE FAMILY

It combines well with Eucalyptus, Lavender, Rosemary, Grapefruit, Dill, Carrot, Marjoram, Savory, Basil, Niaouli, Sweet Thyme, Pine, Anise, Sage, Cinnamon, Clove and Ravensara.

Major Chemical Constituents: menthol, menthone, menthyle acetate, β caryophellene, neomenthol, 1, 8-cineole.

The aroma is fresh, bright, penetrating and minty. Peppermint is steam distilled. The parts used in the extracting of this essence are the leaves, flowers and tops. Peppermint is colorless.

Circulatory System: Varicose veins, palpitations. *External Use:* Massage, reflexology, acupressure.

Digestive System: Nausea, vomiting, colic, flatulence, indigestion, gallstones, bile blockage, beneficial for the stomach and the liver. *Internal Use:* Orally 2 to 5 drops in the Solubol™ with water three times daily.

Immune System: Warming and stimulating properties are particularly valuable at the onset of a cold, sinus problems, shingles. It makes a blend more dynamic and always acts as a general tonic and immune stimulant. Anti-infectious, antiviral, bactericidal, pulmonary, tuberculosis and feverish conditions. *External Use:* Massage, diffuse, reflexology, acupressure, spritzer. *Internal Use:* Orally 2 to 5 drops in Solubol™ with water three times daily.

Intestinal System: Gastric ulcers, constipation, diarrhea, flatulence, hemorrhoids and parasites. *External Use:* Ointment massage. *Internal Use:* Orally 2 to 5 drops in Solubol™ with water three times daily.

Mind System: Mental fatigue, shock, helplessness, overwork, sluggishness, lethargy, apathy, depression, anxiety and addictions. It's clarifying, awakening, stimulating, penetrating, regenerating, emotionally refreshing and improves concentration and vitality. *External Use:* Massage, diffuse, reflexology, acupressure, spritzer. *Internal Use:* Orally 2 to 5 drops in Solubol™ with water three times daily.

Nervous System: Headaches, migraines, shingles, shock, and hypertension. *External Use:* Massage, reflexology, acupressure, sprizter.

Reproductive System: Uterine tonic, hot flashes, impotence, P.M.S, for breast engorgement, labor pains, and lack of period. *External Use:* Massage, compress, inhalation. *Internal Use:* Orally 2 to 5 drops in Solubol™ with water three times daily.

Respiratory System: Sinus, expectorant for bronchioles, pulmonary tuberculosis, asthma. *External Use:* Inhalation, diffuse, massage. *Internal Use:* Orally 2 to 5 drops in Solubol™ with water three times daily.

Skeletal System: Sciatica, rheumatism, joint pain, and muscle pain. *External Use:* Massage, acupressure, reflexology, compress.

Skin and Hair Systems: Bruises, canker sores, skin that is swollen, acne, sunburn, insectbites, and athlete's foot. *External Use:* Ointment, diffuse, massage, clay.

Urinary System: Infection of the kidneys. *Internal Use:* Orally 2 to 5 drops in Solubol™ with water three times daily.

Contraindications: Do not use during first 16 weeks of pregnancy. Skin irritant. Do not use on Children under 2 years of age.

Pine

(Pinus sylvestris)
COUNTRY OF ORIGIN: Austria
CONFEREE FAMILY

It combines well with Clary Sage, Cypress, Lavender, Tea Tree, Rosemary, Juniper, Lemon, Grapefruit, Eucalyptus, Frankincense, Marjoram, Peppermint, Bergamot, Ravensara, Cedarwood, Sandalwood and Sweet Thyme.

Major Chemical Constituents: α and β pinene, limonene, Δ 3 carene.

The aroma is a strong, fresh, balsamic, pine odor. Pine is steam distilled. The parts used in extracting the essence are the branches. Pine is colorless.

Circulatory System: Stimulates circulation. *External Use:* Put a small amount of pine in an oil or ointment and massage on the area.

Glandular System: Toning and restorative to the adrenal glands. *Internal Use:* Orally use 3 to 5 drops in Solubol™ with water three times daily.

Immune System: Germicidal. *External Use:* Diffuse, massage, reflexology.

Mind System: Guilt, punishing yourself, acceptance, understanding, worry, exhaustion. *External Use:* Diffuse, inhalation, bath, put a small amount of pine in an oil and massage on the area.

Muscular System: Warming to the muscles helping with fatigue and pain. *External Use:* Put a small amount of pine in an oil or ointment and massage on the area.

Reproductive System: Impotence, prostatitis. *Internal Use:* Orally use 3 to 5 drops in Solubol™ with water three times daily.

Respiratory System: Expectorant for coughs, asthma, bronchial infections, sinus, pulmonary tuberculosis, air disinfectant, antiseptic, good to diffuse during cold and flu season, anti-infectious. *External Use:* Diffuse, bath, steam inhalation. *Internal Use:* Orally 3 to 5 drops in Solubol™ with water three times daily.

Skeletal System: Rheumatism and gout. *External Use:* Put a small amount of pine in an oil or ointment and massage on the area, bath, reflexology.

Urinary System: Prostatitis, infection of the bladder. *Internal Use:* Orally 3 to 5 drops in Solubol™ with water three times daily.

Contraindications: Can irritate the skin; take care when using it in the bath.

Ravensara

(Ravensara aromatica)
COUNTRY OF ORIGIN: Malaysia
LAURACEAE FAMILY
It combines well with Bergamot, Tea Tree, Black Pepper, Frankincense, Ginger, Sweet Thyme, Sandalwood, Red Thyme, Cedarwood, Roman Chamomile and Lavender.

Major Chemical Constituents: 1, 8 cineole, α terpineol, terpineol 4-01.

The aroma is soft and subtle. Ravensara is steam distilled. The parts used in extracting the essence are the young leafy twigs. In Malaysian language, Ravensara means "the tree with good leaves."

Immune System: Antiviral, fevers, chills, shivers, viral hepatitis, viral infections, flus, colds, measles. *External Use:* Diffuse, bath, compress, inhalation, massage. *Internal Use:* Orally 2 to 3 drops in Solubol™ with water twice daily.

Mind System: It helps one to want to live to attain their goals. *External Use:* Diffuse, bath, compress, inhalation, massage.

Muscular System: Muscle stress and pain. *External Use:* Diffuse, bath, compress, inhalation, massage.

Nervous System: Nervous fatigue, depression, anxiety, lethargy. *External Use:* Diffuse, bath, compress, inhalation, massage.

Reproductive System: Genital herpes. *External Use:* Diffuse, bath, compress, inhalation, massage.

Respiratory System: Bronchitis, sinus, whooping cough, tuberculosis. *External Use:* Compress, bath, massage, diffuse, inhalation. *Internal Use:* Orally 2 to 3 drops in Solubol™ with water twice daily.

Skeletal System: Rheumatoid arthritis. *External Use:* Compress, massage, bath, inhalation.

Skin System: Shingles, acne, chicken pox, measles. *External Use:* Diffuse, bath, compress, inhalation, massage.

Contraindications: None.

Red Thyme

(Thymus vulgaris)
COUNTRY OF ORIGIN: Spain
LABIATAE FAMILY
It combines well with Lemon, Tea Tree, Rosemary, Eucalyptus, Pine, Cypress, Lavender, Juniper, Sage, Oregano, Peppermint and Clove.

Major Chemical Constituents: thymol, carvacrol.

The aroma is sharp and woody. Red thyme is steam distilled. The parts used in extracting the essence are the leaves and flowering tops. The color is an orange red to a grayish brown.

Circulatory System: Raises blood pressure, stimulates circulation, purification of the blood, stimulates the lymphatic system, cellulite and obesity. *External Use:* Massage.

Digestive System: Stomach viruses. *Internal Use:* Orally 2 to 3 drops in Solubol™ with water twice daily for ten days.

Immune System: Bactericidal, antiseptic, antibiotic, whooping cough, earaches, pulmonary tuberculosis, flu originating from the chills, colds and sinus infection. It stimulates the immune system and spleen. *Internal Use:* Orally 2 to 3 drops in Solubol™ with water twice daily for ten days.

Intestinal System: Parasites and intestinal viruses. *Internal Use:* Orally 2 to 3 drops in Solubol™ with water twice daily for ten days.

Mind System: Stimulates the mind, mental clarity, sharpness, courage, stamina, uplifting for depression. *External Use:* Massage, compress, clay pack.

Nervous System: Stimulates the nervous system. *External Use:* Massage, compress, reflexology, acupressure.

Reproductive System: Vaginitis. *Internal Use:* Orally 2 to 3 drops in Solubol™ with water twice daily for ten days.

Respiratory System: Sinus infection, bronchitis, expectorant, pulmonary tuberculosis ,whooping cough, colds. *External Use:* Inhalation. *Internal Use:* Orally 10 drops in Solubol™ with water three times daily for ten days.

Skeletal System: Arthritis, rheumatism. *External Use:* Massage, reflexology, compress.

Skin and Hair Systems: Abscesses, boils, scars. *External Use:* Compresses, massage.

Urinary System: Stimulates the kidneys, helps with excretion and kidney infections. *Internal Use:* Orally 2 to 3 drops in Solubol™ with water twice daily for ten days.

Contraindications: Do not use during pregnancy. Skin irritant. Toxic in high doses; only use red thyme orally for ten days.

Roman Chamomile

(Athemis nobilis)
COUNTRY OF ORIGIN: France
COMPOSITAE FAMILY
It combines well with Lavender, Bergamot, Geranium, Thyme, Rose, Nutmeg, Jasmine, Cedar, Lemon, Clary Sage, Mandarin, Dill, Orange, Neroli, Basil, Cinnamon, Ginger, Tangerine and Oregano.

Major Chemical Constituents: isobutyl angelate, isomyle, isoamyl angelate.

The aroma is sweet, earthy, warm, herby, tart and apple-like. Roman chamomile is steam distilled. The parts used in the extracting of this essence are the flowers and leaves. It is colorless. Roman chamomile is excellent for children.

Circulatory System: Anemia. *Internal Use:* Orally 2 to 3 drops in Solubol™ with water.three times daily.

Digestive System: Stimulates the liver and spleen, colic, bloating, gas and indigestion. *External Use:* Massage, bath, acupressure, reflexology, compress. *Internal Use:* Orally 2 to 3 drops in Solubol™ with water.

Immune System: Aantibacterial, antiseptic, disinfectant, earaches, ear infections, eye infections, fevers, antiviral. *External Use:* Massage, compress, reflexology, eye wash. *Internal Use:* Orally 2 to 3 drops in Solubol™ with water twice daily.

Intestinal System: Diarrhea. *Internal Use:* Douche, suppositories, gargle, Orally 2 to 3 drops in Solubol™ with water three times daily.

Mind System: Calming effect on hysteria and emotions like anger, fretfulness, worry and short temper. It also relaxes and appeases the emotions. *External Use:* Diffuse, compress, massage, reflexology. *Internal Use:* Orally 2 to 3 drops in Solubol™ with water three times daily.

Nervous System: Calms, soothes, relaxes and helps with insomnia, headaches, and anorexia, as well as tranquilizer withdrawls. *External Use:* Massage, reflexology, acupressure, bath, sniff, diffuse.

Reproductive System: Menstrual problems, vaginitis, menopausal problems. *Internal Use:* Douche, suppositories, orally 2 to 3 drops in Solubol™ with water twice daily.

Respiratory System: Asthma, hay fever, congestion. *External Use:* Diffuse, compress, massage. *Internal Use:* Orally 2 to 3 drops in Solubol™ with water three times daily.

Skeletal System: Inflammation of joints, strains, sprains, dull aches, teething, toothaches, rheumatism. *External Use:* Diffuse, facial compress, massage, inhalation. *Internal Use:* For teething, 1 drop in water or Aloe Vera gel on cotton ball and place on area where teething.

Skin and Hair Systems: Boils, abscesses, burns, oily or dry skin, sunburns, eczema, psoriasis, wounds, antiseptic properties, for highlights in blonde hair. It is used in many shampoos. *External Use:* Massage, inhalation, diffuse, facial compress, clay packs, shampoo.

Urinary System: Infection of the bladder and kidneys. *External Use:* Compress, reflexology, massage. *Internal Use:* Orally 2 to 3 drops in Solubol™ with water twice daily.

Contraindications: Do not use during pregnancy.

Rose Bulgarian

(Rosedamascenas p. miller)
COUNTRY OF ORIGIN: Bulgaria
ROSACEAE FAMILY
It combines well with Nutmeg, Jasmine, Sandalwood, Neroli, Geranium, Bergamot, Ylang Ylang, Clary Sage and all citrus.

Major Chemical Constituents: citronellol, geraniol, nonadecane, nerol, phenethyl alcohol.

The aroma is rich, warm, floral and spicy. This is one of the two essential oils that can be used in every aspect of aromatherapy. Rose Bulgarian can be used spiritually, emotionally, medicinally and in perfumery. The color is pale yellow to an orangish-yellow.

Circulatory System: Regulates the heart, increases circulation. *External Use:* Massage, compress, bath, diffuse.

Digestive System: Liver, stomach, lowers cholesterol. *Internal Use:* Orally 2 to 3 drops in Solubol™ with water twice daily.

Immune System: Antibacterial, antiviral, anti-infectious, good for colds, sore throats. *External Use:* Massage, reflexology. *Internal Use:* Orally 2 to 3 drops in Solubol™ with water three times daily. Gargle.

Mind System: Rose is one of the most emotionally balancing of essential oils. It helps to alleviate anger, sadness, grief and depression. Rose brings out the strength and courage to overcome, to reach deep into recesses of the heart. *External Use:* Massage, inhalation, compress, reflexology, diffusion, bath.

Nervous System: Shingles, migraine. *External Use:* Massage, bath, diffuse, eye compress.

Reproductive System: Tones the uterus, stimulates menstruation, increases vaginal secretions, acts as an aphrodisiac, may increase sperm count, and helps with infertility, vaginitis, herpes, and childbirth. *External Use:* Massage, bath, diffuse, compress, reflexology. *Internal Use:*

Orally 2 to 3 drops with Solubol™ and water twice daily. Douche.
Skin System: Eczema, dry skin, wound healing because of its antiseptic properties and anti-infectious qualities, conjunctivitis, scarring, shingles. *External Use:* Facial, massage, compress, ointment.

Contraindications: None.

Rosemary

(Rosemarinus officinalis)
COUNTRY OF ORIGIN: Morocco, Tunesia.
LABIATAE FAMILY
It combines well with Peppermint, Sage, Bergamot, Swiss Pine, Grapefruit, Lemon, Juniper, Basil, Clary Sage, Hyssop, Lavender, Frankincense, Oregano, Cedar, Clove and Chamomile.

Major Chemical Constituents: 1,8 cineol, camphre, pinenes.

The aroma is strong, woody and camphoric. Rosemary is steam distilled. The parts used in extracting the essence are the flowers and twigs. The color is a clear to a pale yellow.

Circulatory System: Raises blood pressure and is used for cold hands and feet, varicose veins, anemia and a heart tonic. *External Use:* Massage, reflexology, bath. *Internal Use:* Orally 3 to 4 drops in Solubol™ with water two to three times daily.
Digestive System: Liver ailments, gallbladder, increases secretion of bile, gallstones, gout, indigestion, cirrhosis, jaundice, diabetes, cholesterol. *External Use:* Massage, compress. *Internal Use:* Orally 3 to 4 drops in Solubol™ with water two to three times.
Glandular System: Lowers sugar levels in diabetics. *External Use:* Reflexology, bath, acupressure, massage. *Internal Use:* Orally 3 to 4 drops in Solubol™ with water two to three times daily.
Immune System: Flu, colds, coughs, anti-fungal, antiseptic, earaches, whooping cough and catarrh. *External Use:* Massage, compress. *Internal Use:* Orally 3 to 4 drops in Solubol™ with water two to three times daily.

Intestinal System: Constipation, intestinal infection, colitis, diaherra, gas. *External Use:* Massage, compress. *Internal Use:* Orally 2 to 3 drops in Solubol™ with water three times daily.

Mind System: For depression, sluggishness, mental fatigue, poor memory, mental strain, nerve tonic, brain stimulant, weak ego, apathy, mood swings. Stimulates the central nervous system. *External Use:* Diffuse, massage.

Nervous System: Headaches, migraines, for people who have partially lost their senses of smell, speech, sight, taste, or touch. Stimulates the nervous system, and helps fight fatigue and paralysis. *External Use:* Diffuse, inhalation, bath, compress, massage, reflexology, acupressure. *Internal Use:* Orally 3 to 4 drops in Solubol™ with water two to three times daily.

Reproductive System: Relieving cramps, stimulates menstruation, leucorrhea and regulates ovarian function. *External Use:* Reflexology, compress, acupressure, massage. *Internal Use:* Orally 3 to 4 drops in Solubol™ with water two to three times daily.

Respiratory System: Asthma, cold, earaches, whooping coughs, coughs and sinus. *External Use:* Diffuse, acupressure, compress, inhalation, massage. *Internal Use:* Orally 3 to 4 drops in Solubol™ with water two to three times daily.

Skeletal System: Tendinitis, muscular pain, sprains. *External Use:* Bath, massage, reflexology, acupressure.

Skin and Hair Systems: For oily skin, acne, blemished skin and brings out red highlights in brunettes. *External Use:* Facials, massage, diffuse, compresses, clay packs, shampoo.

Urinary System: Bed-wetting, diuretic. *Internal Use:* Orally 3 to 4 drops in Solubol™ with water two to three times daily.

Contraindications: If you are pregnant, epileptic or have high blood pressure, do not use this oil.

Sandalwood

(Santalum album)

COUNTRY OF ORIGIN: India, New Calendonia.

SANTALACEAE FAMILY

It combines well with Frankincense, Geranium, Grapefruit, Clary Sage, Palmarosa, Ylang Ylang, Lavender, Roman Chamomile, Rose, Jasmine, Cinnamon, Patchouli, Bergamot, Ginger, Nutmeg, Clove and Benzoin.

Major Chemical Constituents: α santalene, α santalola, β santalene, β santalol.

The aroma is warm, woody, sweet, spicy, oriental and soft balsamic. Sandalwood is steam distilled. The parts used for extracting the essential oil are the roots and the heartwoods. Sandalwood is one of the oldest known perfume materials, and it has at least 4,000 years of history and uninterrupted use. The color is pale yellow to a yellow.

Digestive System: Calming to the stomach, antispasmodic. *External Use:* Bath, massage, reflexology, acupressure.

Immune System: Antibacterial, antiseptic. *Internal Use:* Orally 2 to 3 drops in Solubol™ with water three times daily.

Intestinal System: Gastritis, diarrhea. *External Use:* Massage, reflexology, ointment. *Internal Use:* Orally 2 to 3 drops in Solubol™ with water three times daily.

Mind System: Calming, soothing, sedative, comforting, uplifting and grounding. For isolation and depression. *External Use:* Bath, massage, reflexology, acupressure.

Muscular System: Relieve muscle spasms. *External Use:* Massage, compress.

Nervous System: Insomnia, depression. *External Use:* Massage, bath, reflexology.

Reproductive System: An aphrodisiac that helps with impotence, prostatitis, menstrual cramps, frigidity and gonorrhea. *Internal Use:* Orally 2 to 3 drops in Solubol™ with water three times daily.

Respiratory System: An expectorant for bronchitis, sinus, laryngitis and sore throat. *External Use:* Massage, reflexology. *Internal Use:* Orally

2 to 3 drops in Solubol™ with water three times daily. For a sore throat use as a gargle.

Skin System: An antiseptic that regenerates tissue and relieves acne, dry skin, scarring and skin infections. Also used in hair care and perfumes. *External Use:* Facial, compress, massage.

Urinary System: Diuretic for infection of the bladder. *Internal Use:* Orally 2 to 5 drops in Solubol™ with water three times daily.

Contraindications: None

Spikenard

(Nardostachys jatamansi)
COUNTRY OF ORIGIN: India, Japan
It combines well with Pine, Rose, Cedarwood, Frankincense, Myrrh, Neroli, Lavender, Patchouli, Vetiver, Geranium and Palma Rosa.

Major Chemical Constituents: caraene, seychellene, α patchoulene, β patchoulene, patchoulol, β -ionone.

The aroma is a sweet, heavy, woody and spicy animal odor. The dried root is steam distilled. The color is a pale yellow to an amber.

Circulatory System: Heart palpitations. *External Use:* Massage, reflexology, compress, acupressure, bath.

Intestinal System: Hemorrhoids. *External Use:* Ointment, Sitz bath, compresses.

Mind System: Relieves emotional tension and insomnia. *External Use:* Massage, reflexology, compress, acupressure, bath.

Nervous System: Insomnia, headache, indigestion caused by nervousness, physical tension. *External Use:* Massage, bath, inhalation.

Skeletal System: Backache. *External Use:* Massage.

Skin System: For dry or mature skin, rashes and psoriasis. Excellent for inflammation. *External Use:* Compresses, inhalation, bath, ointment.

Contraindications: None

Sweet Marjoram

(Origanum marjorana)
COUNTRY OF ORIGIN: Spain, France
LABIATAE FAMILY
It combines well with Pine, Rosemary, Tea Tree, Sweet Thyme, Lavender, Cypress, Roman Chamomile, Basil, Bergamot, Black Pepper, Clary Sage, Fennel, Juniper, Lemon, Orange and Peppermint.

Major Chemical Constituents: terpinene 4 ol, cis and trans, thujanol 4.

The aroma is warm, spicy, aromatic, camphoric and woody. Sweet marjoram is steam distilled. The parts used in the extracting of the essence are the leaves and flowering tops. The color is a pale yellow to amber.

Circulatory System: Helps to normalize blood pressure. *Internal Use:* Orally 2 to 3 drops in Solubol™ with water twice daily.

Digestive System: Calming to the stomach, allowing for better digestion. *Internal Use:* Orally 2 to 3 drops in Solubol™ with water twice daily.

Immune System: Antiviral, antibacterial, ear infection and antifungal. *External Use:* Compress, massage, reflexology.

Intestinal System: Gas, parasites, constipation. *External Use:* Massage, compress, reflexology, acupressure. *Internal Use:* Orally 3 to 4 drops in Solubol™ and water three times daily.

Mind System: Anxiety, confusion, fear, forgetfulness, impatience, instability. *External Use:* Compress, massage, reflexology.

Muscular System: It's analgesic properties make it beneficial to painful stiff muscles. *External Use:* Massage, compress, diffuse, reflexology.

Nervous System: Anxiety, insomnia, migraines, nervous debility, mental instability, stress from work. *External Use:* Diffuse, compress, massage, reflexology. *Internal Use:* Orally 3 to 4 drops in Solubol™ with water three times daily.

Reproductive System: For irritation of the genitals and menstrual challenges. *External Use:* Compress, reflexology, massage, ointment.

Respiratory System: Bronchitis, asthma, expectorant. *Internal Use:* Orally 3 to 4 drops in Solubol™ with water three times daily.
Skin System: Bites, burns. *External Use:* Compress, ointment, spritzer.
Urinary System: Cystitis. *Internal Use:* Orally 2 drops in Solubol™ with water four times daily.

Contraindications: None.

Sweet Thyme

(Thyme vulgaris linalool)
COUNTRY OF ORIGIN: France, Spain C.T.
LABIATAE FAMILY
It combines well with Grapefruit, Vetiver, Juniper, Cypress, Geranium, Pine, Roman Chamomile, Eucalyptus, Rosemary, Lemon and Lavender.

Major Chemical Constituents: linalool, paracymene, α terpinene.

The aroma is soft, woody and herby. Sweet thyme is steam distilled. The parts used in the extracting of the essence are the flowering tops.

Circulatory System: Increase circulation, low blood pressure. *External Use:* Massage, bath, reflexology. *Internal Use:* Orally 3 to 5 drops three times daily in Solubol™ with water.
Digestive System: Helps the liver to function, diabetes and bad breath. *Internal Use:* Orally 3 to 5 drops three times daily in Solubol™ with water twice daily.
Immune System: Flu, ear infections, colds. *Internal Use:* Orally 3 to 5 drops in Solubol™ with water twice daily.
Intestinal System: Parasites and infections. *External Use:* Clay, compresses packs. *Internal Use:* Orally 3 to 5 drops in Solubol™ with water three times daily.
Nervous System: Shingles, stress, exhaustion, depression, debility, general fatigue. *External Use:* Bath, massage. *Internal Use:* Orally 3 to 5 drops in Solubol™ with water three time daily.
Reproductive System: For prostatitis, vaginitis, Candida Albicans,

vaginal infections, lack of period, impotence and thick-heavy discharge. *External Use:* Compresses (castor oil). *Internal Use:* Suppositories, douche.

Respiratory System: Relieves bronchitis, tonsillitis, sore throat, coughs, asthma and whooping cough. *External Use:* Diffuse, inhalation, massage, compress, gargle. *Internal Use:* Orally 3 to 5 drops in Solubol™ with water three times daily and suppositories.

Skeletal System: Rheumatism, arthritis. *External Use:* Massage, compress (castor oil).

Skin System: Its antiseptic properties are beneficial to wounds, acne, psoriasis, shingles, insect bites, athlete's foot, fungal infections of the skin, eczema, abscesses and body odor *External Use:* Ointment, compress, bath, clay packs.

Urinary System: Kidney infection. *Internal Use:* Orally 3 to 5 drops in Solubol™ with water three times daily.

Contraindications: Do not use during pregnancy. Safe for children.

Tea Tree

(Melaleuca alternifolia)
COUNTRY OF ORIGIN: Australia
MYRTEACA FAMILY
It combines well with Lavender, Clove, Rosemary, Chamomile, Thyme, Pine, Eucalyptus, Lemon, Orange, Mandarin, Tangerine, Juniper and Cypress.

Major Chemical Constituents: terpinene -4 -01, α terpineol, para-cymene, Y terpineol.

The aroma is spicy, strong, fresh and sharp. Tea tree is steam distilled. The parts used in the extracting of the essence are the leaves. The color is clear to a pale yellowish green.

Immune System: Antiseptic, anti-infectious, antiviral, antifungal, used in first aid kits, sore throats, cold sores, ear aches, ear infections, toothpaste and mouth washes, for its germicidal and solvent properties. It is effective against Candida. To control bacteria in spas and pools. With recent confirmation of Tea Tree oil's dramatic effectiveness against methicillin-resistant Staphylococcus aureus, as published in the *Lancet*, research has now shifted to focus on the potential applications of tea tree oil in hospital wound care treatment. *External Use:* Diffuse, inhalation, massage, bath, compresses, neat, gargle for sore throats.

Mind System: Sluggishness, tiredness, weakness, vigor and cleansing. *External Use:* Diffuse, inhalation, massage, bath, compresses, heat.

Nervous System: Herpes and shingles due to stress. *External Use:* Diffuse, inhalation, massage, bath, compresses, heat.

Reproductive System: Vaginitis, yeast infections, jock itch. *External Use:* Powder, ointment. *Internal Use:* Douche, suppositories.

Skin and Hair Systems: Skin irritation, wounds, sores, athlete's foot, cold sores, gum and mouth ulcers, ring worm, acne, dandruff, rashes, insect and spider bites. Soothing and has topical anesthetic and anti-inflammatory effects. Insect repellent, deodorants, soaps, lotions and shampoo. *External Use:* Diffuse, inhalation, massage, bath, compresses and neat.

Contraindications: None.

Vetiver

(Vetiveria zizanoides)
COUNTRY OF ORIGIN: Haiti
GRAMINACEAE FAMILY
It combines well with Bois de Rose, Cedarwood, Jasmine, Neroli, Petitgrain, Sandalwood, Clary Sage, Patchouli, Rose and Ylang Ylang.

Major Chemical Constituents: α vetiverol, A vetiverol B, α vetivone, khusimol.

The aroma is deep, earthy, woody, sweet and heavy. Vetiver is steam distilled. The parts used for extracting the essence are the roots. The roots come from a grass also grown to protect the soil from eroding on mountainous slopes. The color is amber to a dark brown.

Circulatory System: Stimulating to the circulation. Its toning effects are good for the heart, helps with cold hands and feet. *External Use:* Massage, bath, reflexology, acupressure.

Mind System: Hysteria, depression, repression, guilt, grief. There is a saying, "You are so highly minded, you are no earthly good." Vetiver grounds and balances us so we can do our earthly works. It can be helpful with addictive behavior. It connects us to the earth and brings vital energy to us. *External Use:* Massage, bath, reflexology, acupressure.

Muscular System: Relieves muscle aches and pains. *External Use:* Massage, bath, reflexology, acupressure.

Nervous System: Helps with nervous exhaustion, stress, insomnia and over sensitivity. *External Use:* Massage, bath, reflexology, acupressure.

Reproductive System: Aphrodisiac, P.M.S, frigidity. *External Use:* Massage, bath, reflexology, acupressure.

Skeletal System: Antispasmodic properties help with arthritis pain. *External Use:* Massage, bath, reflexology, acupressure.

Skin System: For oily skin, acne and stretchmarks. Also tones the skin. *External Use:* Facial, massage, bath, reflexology, acupressure.

Contraindications: None

Ylang Ylang

(Canaga odorantissimum)
COUNTRY OF ORIGIN: Madagascar
ANNONANCEAE FAMILY
It combines well with Orange, Bergamot, Rose, Sandalwood, Jasmine, Bois de Rose, Ginger, Nutmeg, Clary Sage, Vetiver and Black Pepper.

Major Chemical Constituents: germacrene, D farnesene, benzyle acetate, linalool, benzyle benzoate, benzyle salicylate.

The aroma is sweet, voluptuous and exotic. Ylang Ylang is steam distilled. The parts used in extracting the essence are the flowers. These yellow flowers are found on trees in the tropics. The color is yellowish.

Circulatory System: Tachycardia (abnormal heart rate), high blood pressure. *External Use:* Massage, compress, bath.

Intestinal System: Intestinal infections. *External Use:* Massage, compress, bath, castor oil pack.

Mind System: Depression, anger, fear, nervous, headaches, inner coldness, frustration, anxiety. Calming for all negative emotions. *External Use:* Massage, reflexology, bath, acupressure, compress.

Nervous System: Calming when over-excited. Acts as a sedative and helps relieve headaches. *External Use:* Bath, massage.

Reproductive System: Well-reputed as an aphrodisiac. For frigidity, P.M.S. and impotence. *External Use:* Bath, massage, compress.

Respiratory System: Helps create rhythmic breathing. *External Use:* Inhalation, massage, bath, compress.

Skin and Hair Systems: Acne, skin disorders which contains pus or form pus. It's moisturizing and rejuvenating to the skin. *Hair care:* helps with split ends and scalp treatment. Antiseptic, perfumes. *External Use:* Perfume, facials, compresses, lotions, hair care, shampoos, clay, inhalation.

Contraindications: Too much can cause headache if too concentrated.

Section 5
Essential Oil Blends

Blend #1 Peppermint, Rosemary, Niaouli and Geranium

Major Chemical Constituents: 1,8 cineole, menthol, citronellol, pine, linalool, camphor.

The aromas of peppermint and rosemary warm and stimulate the respiratory system, opening up the sinuses, bronchioles and lungs. Niaouli, peppermint and geranium's antiseptic properties are good for sinusitis, bronchitis, tonsillitis and sore throats. Niaouli is anti-catarrhal, moving the mucous out of the sinuses, bronchioles and lungs. This blend is also used to warm and stimulate the large intestine.

Respiratory System: Bronchitis, chronic bronchitis, pneumonia, sinusitis, sore throat, tonsillitis and whooping cough. *External Uses:* Massage 230 drops in 1 oz. of massage oil for chronic bronchitis, pneumonia and whooping cough. Or massage 23 drops in 1 oz. of massage oil for sinusitis, bronchitis. Massage the large intestine area, chest, back, lungs and reflex points on the foot that correspond to these organs. It can also be used in compresses for bronchitis, pneumonia, chronic bronchitis, sinusitis, sore throat and tonsillitis. Or in a bath use 10 drops of blend in 1 1/2 t. of Solubol™. Mix thoroughly and put in bath tub. *Internal Use:* Orally 3 to 5 drops in 1 t. of Solubol™ in 4 oz. of water. Gargle 10 drops in 1 1/2 t. of Solubol™ in 4 oz. of water or sore throats and tonsillitis.

Contraindications: Do not use ·during pregnancy, or if you have high blood pressure or asthma.

Blend #2 Niaouli, Geranium, Juniper, Vetiver, Grapefruit, Sweet Thyme, Cypress, Rosemary

Major Chemical Constituents: Limonene, pinene, citronellol, linalool.

Grapefruit, juniper and geranium stimulate the fluids in the body helping it to eliminate the toxins. Rosemary, sweet thyme and vetiver stimulate the circulation. Rosemary increases the secretion of bile to help the gall bladder and liver support digestion. Juniper stimulates the pancreas improving digestion. Grapefruit tones the skin bringing the circulation to the surface of the skin. Cypress also has astringent and toning properties. This blend is excellent to help detox and move the lymphatic system. It is also good for muscular and joint pain.

Digestive System: Indigestion, gout. *External Use:* Massage. *Internal Use:* Orally 2 to 3 drops in 1 t. of Solubol™ in 4 oz. of water three times daily.

Lymphatic System: Swollen glands, cellulite, weight loss. *External Use:* Massage, bath

Mind System: For alcoholism and helps pain for the terminally ill. *External Use:* Bath, massage.

Muscular System: Muscle pain. *External Use:* bath, massage.

Skeletal System: Arthritis. *External Use:* Bath, massage.

Urinary System: Diuretic. *External Use:* Bath, 10 drops in 1 1/2 t. Solubol™ mix in bath water. Massage 23 to 30 drops in massage oil. Massage twice daily.

Contraindications: Do not use if you are pregnant or have chronic kid-ney problems, high blood pressure or epilepsy.

Blend #3 Clary Sage, Geranium, Nutmeg, and Rose Bulgarian

Major Chemical Constituents: Citronellol, linalyl, acetate, sabinene, pinene.

The antispasmodic, warming and relaxing properties of clary sage and nutmeg are helpful for menstrual tension, cramps and lower back pain. Historically, clary sage is used for night sweats and hot flashes during menopause. The queen of essential oils, rose, has long been praised for its balancing qualities for the reproductive system and emotions; gerani-um also shares these qualities. This blend is good for nervous tension, irritability, stress, P.M.S., endometriosis and hot flashes.

Reproductive System: PMS: *External Use:* Diffuse 10 minutes a day for 10 days before menses. Massage 23 to 30 drops in 1 oz. of massage oil for 10 days before menses and during menses. Do this through three cycles, applying daily.

MENSTRUAL CRAMPS: Massage it directly (neat) on the lower abdomen until cramps subside. *Compress:* A warm water compress with 10 drops of #3 Blend on it. Lay on lower abdomen until cramps subside, change when compress becomes cold. *Bath:* 10 drops in 1 1/2 t. of Solubol™ in bath.

HOT FLASHES: *External Use:* Sniff, small, short sniffs directly out of the bottle. Massage 23 to 30 drops in 1 oz. massage oil on lower back lower abdomen twice daily.

ENDOMETROSIS: *External Use:* Massage 230 drops in 1 oz. massage oil before bed for 3 months. Massage on lower abdomen, lower back and reflex points of the feet for the uterus twice daily.

INFERTILITY: *External Use:* Massage 230 drops in 1 oz. massage oil before bed for three months. Massage on lower back, lower abdomen and reflex points of the feet for pineal, pituitary glands, ovaries and uterus.

NERVOUS TENSION, IRRITABILITY, AND STRESS: *External Use:* Massage 23 to 30 drops in 1 oz. of massage oil on chest, back of neck and reflex points on the foot for the spine, neck and heart. *Bath:* 10 drops of blend in 1 1/2 t. Solubol™ in bath. *Diffuse:* 25 drops in diffuser for 10 minutes daily.

Contraindications: Do not use during pregnancy or if suffering from uterine tumors caused by too much estrogen. Also do not use in high doses before driving

Blend #4 Clove, Ginger, Nutmeg.

Major Chemical Constituents: Eugenol, zingiberene, pinene, sabinene, pinene.

The deep penetrating aroma of clove stimulates circulation. The warming properties of ginger help to relieve muscle tension, while the analgesic properties of nutmeg help with muscle and joint pain.

Digestive System: Flatulence, indigestion.

Muscle System: Sprains, leg aches. *External Use:* Massage 23 to 30 drops in 1 oz. of massage oil. Massage on sprain after inflammation has gone down. For leg aches apply to legs twice daily or during acute leg pain.

Skeletal System: Arthritis pain and back pain. *External Use:* Massage 60 drops in 1 oz. of massage oil. Massage on joints twice daily and before bed. For fibromygalia, use 60 drops in 1 oz. of massage oil. Massage on shoulders, neck, back and corresponding reflex points on the feet twice daily.

Contraindications: Do not use during pregnancy or on infants and children under 5.

Blend #5 Grapefruit, Basil, Lavender, and Rosemary

Major Chemical Constituents: Limonene, methylchavicol, linalyl acetate, linalool, 1,8 cineole.

The fresh inspiring aroma of grapefruit clears the mind, while the stimulating properties of rosemary and basil increase the circulation to the brain for focus. Lavender helps to calm the mind. This blend with its clear, calm and focused attributes is beneficial when under stress at work, school, studying or at home when under taking major projects and athletic events.

Mind System: Stress, mental strain, tiredness, confusion, fear, anxiety, mental exhaustion, distraction, poor memory, conflict and jitters. Diffuse: 25 drops for 10 minutes twice daily. Massage: 30 drops in 1 oz. of massage oil on forehead, temples, neck, spine and corresponding reflex points on the feet.

Nervous System: ALZHEIMER'S: *External Use:* Massage 60 drops in 1 oz. of massage oil, apply to forehead, neck and reflex points on foot corresponding to the brain, neck and spine. Diffuse 25 drops for 10 minutes twice daily.

A.D.D.: *External Use:* Massage 25 drops in 1 oz. of massage oil, on forehead, back of neck and ears. If no noticeable results add 5 drops of Peppermint to the 25 drops of the blend in 1 oz. of massage oil.

DYSLEXIA: *External Use:* Massage 25 drops with 20 drops Cosmos flower essence on blend in 1 oz. of massage oil. Add 20 drops of Cosmos Flower Essence. Mix thoroughly. Put on back of neck, forehead and spine.

HEADACHES: *External Use:* Sniff out of the bottle. Put on neat on the temples and back of neck. Massage 40 drops in 1 oz. of massage oil. Diffuse 25 drops for five minutes twice daily.

Contraindications: Do not use during pregnancy, high blood pressure or epilepsy.

Blend #6 Roman Chamomile, Lavender, Ravensara, and Tea Tree.

Major Chemical Constituents: 1,8 cineole, terpinen-4-OL-, linalyl acetate, isobutyl angelate, isoamyl metacrylate.

This blend helps guard against infections as well as help fight an infection when suffering from it. Ravensara is well known for its antiviral properties. Tea tree is anti-infectious, antiviral and anti-fungal. Lavender and Roman chamomile are anti-infectious. Roman chamomile, lavender and tea tree are all antiseptic. These properties make this blend beneficial to the immune, mind, respiratory, muscular and skin system. This blend is especially good for acute inflammation.

Immune System: To prevent infections. *External Use:* Massage 60 drops in 1 oz. once daily; massage on feet, chest and back or diffuse to fight infections and viruses: (colds and flu) Can also diffuse 25 drops in diffuser for 10 minutes twice daily, use 10 drops in 1 T. Solubol™ in bathwater or use in hot or cold compresses (pat, don't massage the 10 drops of oil blend). For shingles or herpes and chicken pox sores, put 1 drop on a cotton ball or Q-tip and put directly on infected area. The following recipes can be used for ear infections:

EAR INFECTION RECIPES
25-30 drops of blend
1 oz massage oil

Combine blend with massage oil and massage on outside ear and mastoid. Or:

1 oz warmed massage oil
25 drops of blend
1 gel capsule of garlic oil

Combine and put two drop inside the ear.
Internal Use: Orally 3 to 5 drops in 1 t. of Solubol™ in 4 ounces of water three times daily; 10 days or use as suppositories.

Mind System: *External Use:* Massage 23 to 30 drops in 1 oz. massage oil on feet and neck. Or diffuse 25 drops in diffuser for 10 minutes twice daily.

Muscular System: Sprains and inflammations. Cold compresses, heat. *External Use:* Massage 30 drops in 1 oz. massage oil on affected areas.

Respiratory System: Dry, hard, spasmodic cough. *External Use:* 12 drops Blend and 7 drops Clary Sage in 1 oz. carrier oil. Massage on chest and back.

Reproductive System: Yeast infections. *Internal Use:* 25 drops in 1 1/2 t. of Solubol™ in 2 quarts of warm water. Suppositories.

Skin System: Cuts. *External Use:* Put it directly on the cut neat. Cold compress.

Contraindications: None.

Blend #7 Roman Chamomile, Mandarin, Lavender, and Rose

Major Chemical Constituents: Limonene, linalyl acetate, terpinene, trans ocimene, isobutyl angelate, isoamyl methacrylate, citronellol.

This blend was especially made for those times when your emotions and mind are saying two different things. The mind keeps racing around with repetitive thoughts of anxiety, fear and worry. The stomach is churning and its difficult to come to a decision about this issue which is what this repetitive thinking is about. Roman Chamomile has long been used for its calming and soothing properties which are helpful to our emotions and digestion. Mandarin is like sunshine to our emotions, it brings light when we are surrounded by dark clouds. Rose strengthens the heart and helps give courage to overcome grief, fear and anger. Universally, lavender is used for its balancing effects when we suffer from anxiety, worry, fretfulness, insomnia and stress.

Digestive System: Colic. *External Use:* Massage 5 drops in 1 oz. of massage oil. Massage stomach and large intestine. Bath: 2 drops in 1/2 t. of Solubol,™ put in water. Acupressure, reflexology, Diffusion.

Intestinal System: Diverticulitis. *External Use:* Massage 75 drops in 1 oz. of massage oil. Massage large intestine in clockwise motion and corresponding reflex points on the feet. Cold compress.

Nervous System: A.D.D: (caused by emotional anxiety). *External Use:* Massage 25 to 30 drops in 1 oz. of massage oil. Put on neck, spine, chest and on corresponding reflex points of foot.

ANXIETY: For worry, fretfulness, stress, panic attack, high blood pressure due to stress and Parkinson's. *External Use:* Bath 10 drops in 1 t. of Solubol™ in the bath water. Diffuse 25 drops for 10 minutes three times daily. Sniff directly from bottle as needed. Massage 25 to 30 drops in 1 oz. of massage oil. Put on stomach, chest, spine, neck and corresponding reflex points on feet.

DEPRESSION: *External Use:* Massage 60 drops in 1 oz. of massage oil. Put on chest, throat, spine and corresponding reflex points on the feet. Bath: 10 drops in 1 1/2 t. of Solubol™ in bath water. Diffuse: 25 drops for 10 minutes three times daily. Sniff.

INSOMNIA: *External Use:* Massage 10 drops in 1 oz. of massage oil. Put on throat, back of neck and reflex points on the feet, and pineal gland reflex. Sniff. Bath.

Reproductive System: P.M.S., postpartum blues, miscarriage and after child birth. *External Use:* Massage 50 drops in 1 ounce of massage oil. Put on chest, back, neck and all of the feet. Bath 20 drops in 2 t. Solubol™ in the bath water. Sitz bath 10 drops in bath water. To help heal the perineum and take down inflammation.

Skin System: Scars and stretchmarks. *External Use:* Massage 25 drops in 1 oz. of olive oil put on stretch marks twice daily.

Contraindications: Photo Toxic.

Blend #8 Sandalwood, Ylang Ylang, Rose Bulgarian, and Jasmine.

Major Chemical Constituents: Santalol, santalol, germacrene, linalool, citronellol, caryophyllene, benzyl benzoate.

This formula was developed to allow us to let go of our daily stresses and to receive and give the intimacy that we all deserve.

For centuries, the aromas of sandalwood, ylang ylang, rose and jasmine have been known for their aphrodisiac qualities. Sandalwood is grounding, allowing us to be present for our loved one. Ylang Ylang is euphoric and calming to negative emotions. Rose helps us to truly give from our hearts. Jasmine is seductive and releases the anxiety, tension and stress that can build up in daily life.

Mind System: Balancing, comforting, relaxing and soothing to anger, sadness, grief, anxiety, depression, fear, frustration and postpartum blues. *External Use:* Massage 23 to 30 drops in 1 oz. of massage oil. Massage on pituitary, pineal, adrenal, ovary, testes, uterus and prostate reflexes on feet. Bath 10 drops 1 1/2 t. Solubol™ in bath water. Sniff three times daily

Reproductive System: FRIGIDITY: *External Use:* Massage 30 drops in massage oil twice daily. Bath 10 drops in 1 1/2 t. of Solubol™ in bath water.

APHRODISIAC: *External Use:* Put 60 drops in massage oil. Massage whole body, reflex points of the pituitary, adrenals, ovaries and testes on the feet. Bath: 10 drops in 1 1/2 t. of Solubol™ in bath water.

IMPOTENCE: *External Use:* Sniff directly from bottle three times daily. Massage on reflex points for the testes, prostate, pituitary, and adrenals. Massage on lower back and lower abdomen.

VAGINAL DRYNESS: *External Use:* Massage 270 drops in l oz. of massage oil or 20 drops in 1 oz. of salve. Massage on lower abdomen, lower back, chest, reflex points on foot pituitary, adrenals, and uterus.

Skin System: DRY SKIN: *External Use:* Put 30 drops in 1 oz. massage oil. Massage where needed. Facial.

PERFUME: *External Use:* Put on neat on lower back, behind the ears, creases of elbows, and behind knees. Spritz.

Contraindications: None

Blend #9 Lavender, Grapefruit, Geranium, and Bergamot.

Major Chemical Constituents: Limonene, linalyl acetate, linalool, citronellol.

The light, citrusy aroma of Grapefruit with the uplifting qualities of Bergamot stimulates the nervous system. Lavender and Geranium are balancing when suffering from mental exhaustion, nervousness, anxiety and restlessness.

Circulatory System: Increases circulation. *External Use:* Massage 60 drops in 1 oz. of massage oil. Massage on after bath or shower. *Bath:* 10 drops in 1 1/2 t. Solubol™ in bath water.

Mind and Nervous System: Mental exhaustion, moodiness, insecurity, tension, irritability, anxiety, worry, hysteria, tiredness and stress due to work or home environment. *External Use:* Sniff directly out of bottle as often as needed. Diffuse 25 drops during work or at home as long as needed. Put 30 drops in 1oz. of massage oil rub on feet and legs.

Skin System: Balancing and toning to the skin (especially oily skin). *External Use:* Facials, massage, compresses and ointments.

Contraindications: Photo Toxic.

Blend #10 Geranium, Roman Chamomile, Rose Bulgarian, Neroli, and Bergamot

Major Chemical Constituents: Citronellol, isobutyl angelate, isoamyl methacrylate, linalool, geraniol, limonene.

The smell of neroli, orange blossoms, transports our minds above the dark clouds of the every day stresses and brings to us the light of the heavens. Deep, earthy and floral is the aroma of the rose from Bulgaria. This aroma is the bridge between the heavens and earth. It is grounding, yet inspirational to the heart. Geranium and Roman chamomile bring their soothing and balancing qualities to this formula. The refreshing aroma of bergamot adds the finishing touch for this blend. This quality is beneficial for anxiety, addictions, depression, stress and tension.

Circulatory System: Hypertension. *External Use:* Sniff, massage and bath.

Intestinal System: Colitis, diarrhea, Irritable Bowel Syndrome and diverticulitis. *External Use:* Massage 270 drops in 1 oz. of massage. Massage on large intestine in clockwise motion and check ileocecal valve. Cold compress.

Mind System: ADDICTIONS, ALCOHOLISM, AND EATING DISORDERS: *External Use:* Sniff as often as needed. Massage 160 drops in 1 oz. of massage oil on neck, spine, liver, pancreas, stomach and do the same reflex points on the feet.

MISCARRIAGE, MENOPAUSAL, ANXIETY, P.M.S.: *External Use:* Massage 23 drops in 1 oz. of massage oil on chest, neck, spine, and corresponding reflex points on feet. Bath 10 drops in 1 1/2 t. of Solubol™ in bath water.

HEART PALPITATIONS(CAUSED BY ANXIETY OR SHOCK): *External Use:* Massage 60 drops in 1 oz. of massage oil. Massage as often as needed on chest, heart, back, on the corresponding reflex points on the foot.

Nervous System: *External Use:* Put 1 drop neat at back of neck. Compress.

Contraindications. None.

Section 6
Ailments A–Z

Key to abbreviations:

(A) ACUPRESSURE
(B) BATH
(C) CLAY COMPRESS
(CO) COLONIC
(D) DIFFUSE
(DO) DOUCHE
(E) ENEMA
(FA) FACIAL
(G) GARGLE
(I) INHALATION
(M) MASSAGE
(N) NEAT
(O) ORAL
(R) REFLEXOLOGY
(S) SITZ BATH
(SP) SUPPOSITORIES

Circulatory System

SINGLE ESSENTIAL OILS

Anemia: Cinnamon, Roman Chamomile, Lemon M, O
Angina: Eucalyptus N, O, M
Blood Pressure, high: Lemon, Lavender, Ylang Ylang, N, M, B, R, A
Blood Pressure, norm: Sweet Marjoram O

Blood Pressure, low: Clove, Hyssop, Rosemary, Red Thyme, Sweet Thyme B, M, R, O

Blood(Purification): Eucalyptus M, C, D, B

Body Temperature(increase): Cistus M, R

Bruising: Helichrysum C, ON, M, B, O

Cellulite: Cedar wood, Red, Thyme, Grapefruit, Juniper, Lemon, Cypress M, R, CL, B

Circulation(increase): Black Pepper, Basil, Dill, Fennel, Red Thyme M,R Lemon, Pine, Rose Bulgarian, Sweet Thyme, Vetiver Cedarwood, Cypress, Juniper M, R, B, C, D Lemongrass O

Circulation(brain): Nutmeg O, Rosemary O, M, B, D, R

Cold Hands, Feet: Rosemary M, R ,B, O, Vetiver M, R, B

Edema: Cistus, Geranium M, B, D Fennel, Lemon O

Heart(calming): Orange M, R, A

Heart(Palpitations): Lavender, Spikenard, Ylang Ylang M, R, C, N, B Peppermint O

Heart(Stimulant): Geranium M, B, D

Heart(tonic): Rosemary O

Heart(irregular heartbeat): Rose Bulgarian, Ylang Ylang M C, B, D

Hemorrhage: Helichrysum O

Obesity: Red Thyme M

Varicose Veins: Cypress, Geranium, Grapefruit, Lemon, Rosemary, Peppermint ON, S, C

Water Retention: Cedarwood M, R, Lemon O

ESSENTIAL OIL BLENDS

Heart Palpitations: Blend #10 M

High blood pressure: Blend #10 D, M

Stimulating: Blend #9 B, D, M

Toning to the Heart: Blend #9 B,D,M

Circulatory System Testimonies

STROKE–HAZEL TILLEY

About 8 years ago, my close friend called me around 10:00 p.m. on a Saturday evening. Her 71 year old mother had suffered a stroke. She asked me if I would come over and help with her mother's condition.

When I arrived, her mother was unable to speak or move the left side of her body. I brought with me 2 vitamin E 400 I.U. capsules, powdered vitamin C drink (1,000 mg per t), 2 CO Q-10 capsules, liquid capsicum extract, 2 garlic oil capsules, liquid hawthorn extract, Rescue Remedy flower essence, olive flower essence, hombeam flower essence, Lavendula Augustifolia essential oil, liquid lobelia extract, 3 magnesium tablets (250 mg each) and 6 oz olive oil.

Immediately I mixed 1/2 t. liquid Lobelia extract, 1/2 t .Capsicum, 1 t. liquid Hawthorn, 20 drops Rescue Remedy and 40 drops of Lavendula Augustifolia in 4 oz. of Olive oil. This mixture was applied to her left ring finger, behind her neck, and then on the reflexology points on her feet corresponding to her heart, adrenals, thyroid, and kidneys. I applied this liquid mixture every 5 minutes. After 20 minutes she could open her mouth and make some sounds. At this time I began administering 1/4 t. Lobelia, 1/4 t. Capsicum, and 4 drops Rescue Remedy to her orally, every 5 minutes. Twenty minutes later we could make out some things she was saying. I then mixed up 1 t. of the vitamin C drink in 4 oz. of water, 2 Vitamin E capsules, 2 CO Q-10 capsules, and three crushed tablets of Magnesium. This mixture was administered in 1 ml. doses orally, every 5 minutes.

In between giving the oral remedies, I mixed 20 drops of Lavender, 20 drops Olive flower essence and 20 drops of Hornbeam in 2 oz. of Olive oil. My sister, a certified reflexologist, arrived and applied this mixture to her feet while I did the points on her hands and head. After 3 hours, she was able to speak more coherently and move the left side of her body.

The next morning, she was better. She ate only potassium broth for the next few days. Within 2 weeks she was back home in Utah taking care of herself. This woman is still alive today and has no signs of having a stroke.

HIGH BLOOD PRESSURE—SOPHIE THEDY
I have used Orange, Lavendula angustifolia, Jasmine grandiflora, and Rose Bulgarian essential oils blended in massage oil for clients with high

blood pressure. For daytime inhalation, this massage blend was applied to the palms of the hands and around the collarbone. When applied on the chest at night, these oils have a lasting effect.

I also suggested that these clients use Blend #10 in a diffuser when going to sleep and upon waking in the morning and that they follow an herbal formula of capsicum, garlic and parsley. They also took lemon juice and capsicum tincture daily to help detox the blood.

This combination of essential oils and herbs regulated the blood pressure of my clients so that they were able to discontinue their medication.

Digestive System

SINGLE OILS
Abdominal(Bloating): Roman Chamomile A, B, C, M, O, R
Abdominal Cramps: Fennel, Hyssop O
Digestion(aids): Basil, Fennel, Grapefruit, Lemongrass O Myrrh B, I, M, R Nutmeg C, M, O Neroli, Peppermint, Ginger, Geranium, Clary Sage B, C, M, O
Digestion(slow): Hyssop O
Anorexia: Bergamot, Fennel, Ginger B, D, M, O
Anti-emetic: Orange, Ginger, Lemon, Peppermint C, M, O
Anti-spasmodic Stomach: Cinnamon O, Sandalwood A, B, M, R
Appetite(stimulant): Bergamot, Fennel, Ginger, Juniper, Hyssop O
Cholesterol Lower: Rose Bulgarian, Rosemary O
Cirrhosis: Juniper, Rosemary O
Colic: Roman Chamomile, Fennel, Neroli, Peppermint C, M, R
Diabetes: Eucalyptus, Geranium, Rosemary, Sweet Thyme O
Gall Bladder: Geranium C, M, Lemon, Rosemary A, C, M, O, R
Gall Stones(dissolve): Eucalyptus, Lemon, Nutmeg, Rosemary O
Gastritis: Roman Chamomile, Clove, Fennel A, C, M, O, R, Lavender C, M
Gastric Ulcers: Peppermint O
Gout: Rosemary C, M, O
Indigestion: Roman Chamomile, Juniper, Peppermint A, C, M, O, R

Internal Bleeding: Cypress, Lemon O

Jaundice: Lemon, Rosemary C, M ,O

Liver: Roman Chamomile, Helichrysum, Lemon, Rose Bulgarian, Rosemary,
Sweet

Thyme: Peppermint C, M

Motion Sickness: Ginger A, C ,M, O, R

Nausea: Fennel, Ginger, Peppermint A, C, M, O, R

Over-indulgence: Orange, Peppermint, Ginger C, O

Pancreas: Juniper A, O, R

Slow Digestion: Hyssop O

Spleen: Roman Chamomile, Fennel, Neroli A, C, M, O, R

Stimulates Appetite: Bergamot, Fennel, Hyssop, Juniper O

Stomach(antispasmodic): Cinnamon O, Sandalwood A, B, M, R

Stomach (neutralizes acid): Black Pepper, Clary Sage, Orange, Sweet Marjoram,
Lemon O

Stomach Distention: Hyssop O

Stomach Infection: Clove O

Stomach Odors: Lemon O

Stomach Virus: Red Thyme O

Stomach Warming: Ginger O

Ulcers: Lavender M

Ulcers(gastric): Peppermint C

Vomiting: Ginger, Lemon, Orange, Peppermint A, C, O, R

BLENDS

Colic: Blend #7 A, B, C, D, M, R

Diabetes: Blend #2, addition Juniper for acute pancreatitis M, O

Indigestion: Blend #2 M, O

Weight Loss: Blend #2 B, M

Gout: Blend #2 M, O

Digestive System Testimony

INGESTION—KARLA CEDARLEAF

I'm always trying new things to eat. On my way to Lorrie's to pick up
my herbs, I stopped at Jack-in-the-Box and got a stuffed chili pepper
with cheese. I arrived at Lorrie's with severe heart burn and gas. She
asked me if I would like to rub some Roman Chamomile, Dill, Lavender,

and Mandarin Orange essential oils on my stomach. I applied them and within minutes my heartburn cleared up.

Glandular System

Adrenals: Basil, Geranium, Pine, Red Thyme A, M, R Pine O
Blood Sugar(balance): Fennel O
Blood Sugar Diabetes(lower): Rosemary, Red Thyme, Eucalyptus O
Glands(stimulate): Cistus D, M, R
Hypoglycemia: Eucalyptus, Fennel O
Pituitary: Sandalwood B, C, D, M
Thyroid: Myrrh M, R

Immune System

SINGLE OILS

Antibacterial: Helichrysum, Patchouli, Pine, B, C, D, M, R Orange, Rose Bulgarian, Sandalwood, Sweet Marjoram, Red Thyme, Tea Tree, Lemongrass, Clary Sage Geranium A, B, C, D, M ,O, R Myrrh B, I, M, ON, R, SP
Antibiotic: Roman Chamomile, Geranium B, C, D, I, M, O Bergamot, Orange, Red Thyme, Cinnamon O, Bois de Rose B, E, M, SP, Lavender A, C, I, M, R
Antifungal: Cedarwood, Patchouli, Myrrh B, C, M, ON, R, Rosemary, Sweet Marjoram, Tea Tree C, M, O, ON
Anti-infection: Frankincense, Sandalwood, Patchouli, Sweet Marjoram, Pine A, C, D, I, M, R, Lemon, Tea Tree, Geranium, RomanChamomile, Rose Bulgarian A, B, C, M, O, R, Clary Sage Helichrysum, Lemongrass, Black Pepper, Red Thyme, Cinnamon, Clove O
Antimicrobial: Black Pepper, Helichrysum, Lemon O
Antiseptic: Roman Chamomile, Clove, Geranium, Grapefruit, Lemon, Sandalwood, Juniper, Orange, Peppermint, Tea Tree B, C, D, I, M, ON, R
Antiviral: Roman Chamomile, Lemon, Rose Bulgarian, Tea Tree, Ravensara C, D, DO, E, G, I, M, O Red Thyme, Cinnamon, Clove C, D, G, I, M, O, Patchouli, Sweet Marjoram A, B, C, M, R
Candida: Eucalyptus, Bois de Rose, Tea Tree, Niaouli, Neroli, Myrrh, Sweet

Thyme A, B, C, DO, E, M, O, ON, R, SP

Catarrh: Rosemary, Eucalyptus A, B, C, G, I, M, ON

Chicken Pox: Bergamot, Cistus, Eucalyptus, Cypress B, C, N, ON

Chills: Ginger, Ravensara B, C, M, R, Red Thyme O

Colds: Frankincense, Sandalwood, Patchouli, Sweet Marjoram, Pine A, C, D, I, M, R, Lemon, Tea Tree, Geranium, Roman Chamomile, Eucalyptus, Rose Bulgarian A, B, C, I, M, O, R, SP, Clary Sage Helichrysum, Lemongrass, Black Pepper, Red Thyme, Cinnamon, Clove O

Cold Sores: Eucalyptus, Tea Tree, Geranium, Lemongrass, Bergamot, Lavender C, CL, N, ON

Coughs: Rosemary, Eucalyptus C, D, I, M, ON, R, SP

Dental Infection(abscess): Clove C, N, ON

Ear Infections: Roman Chamomile, Sweet Thyme, Niaouli, Sweet Marjoram, Tea Tree, Eucalyptus, Lavender, Rosemary

EAR INFECTION RECIPE
    4 drops Roman Chamomile essential oil
    4 drops Lavender essential oil
    6 drops Tea Tree essential oil
    2 drops Sweet Thyme
    1 oz. carrier oil
    1 soft gel capsule of garlic oil

In a small pan, mix essential oils, carrier oil, and garlic oil. Warm on stove to body temperature. Put in 1oz. amber bottle with dropper. Squeeze 1/2 dropperful of this mixture into ear and cover with cotton ball.

Eye Infections: Roman Chamomile

EYE WASH RECIPE
    2 drops Roman Chamomile essential oil
    1/8 t. Solubol ™
    2oz. water

In a small container, mix essential oil Solubol™, and water. Place cotton ball in water and rub it across the eye from inside to outside.

Fevers: Lavender, Basil, Bergamot, Bois de Rose, Ravensara, Ginger B, C, E, M, R, SP Helichrysum, Lemongrass O

Flu: Bergamot, Bois de Rose, Eucalyptus, Frankincense, Lemon, Grapefruit, Ginger, Rosemary, Peppermint, Roman Chamomile, Cypress B, C, D, M

Recovery: Cypress, Eucalyptus, Fennel, Hyssop, Red Thyme, Helichrysum O

Protection against flu: Lavender, Lemon, Niaouli, Peppermint, Pine, Rosemary, Sweet Thyme D, IN, M

Germicidal: Tea Tree, Pine D, I, ON

Gonorrhea: Lemon DO, ON, SP

Hepatitus(viral): Ravensara, Roman Chamomile, Lemon, Rosemary, Peppermint C, M, O

Herpes(Genital: Simplex II): Juniper, Lavender, Sandalwood B, C, M, N, ON

Herpes(zoster-chicken pox): Bergamot, Geranium, Lemon B, C, M, N, ON

Herpes(zoster- shingles): Geranium, Neroli, Lemon, Lemongrass, Peppermint, Ravensara, Roman Chamomile, Lavender, Bergamot B, C, M, N, ON Lemongrass O

Infections: See all essential oils that are bactericidal

Malaria: Eucalyptus, Lemon O

Measles(prevention): Cistus, Eucalyptus, Ravensara, Cypress, C, M, R

Scarlet Fever(prevention): Eucalyptus M, R

Sinus: Eucalyptus, Lavender, Lemon, Niaouli, Peppermint, Pine A, B, C, D, I, M, Red Thyme O

Sore Throat: Geranium, Lemon, Rose Bulgarian, Tea Tree, Ginger G, M, ON

Syphilis: Lemon B, C, N, ON, SP

Terminally Ill: Lavender B, D, I, M, N, ON, R, S

Tuberculosis(pulmonary): Eucalyptus, Lemon, Lavender, Niaouli, Peppermint B, D, I, M, N, ON, SP, Red Thyme, Oregano, Hyssop, Clove, Garlic O

Viral Hepatitis: Ravensara, Roman Chamomile, Lemon, Rosemary, Red Thyme O

Viral Infections: Ravensara(see anti-viral)

White Blood Cells(increase): Cistus C, M, R, Lemon O

Whooping Cough(relieve symptoms): Cistus, Basil, Lavender B, C, D, I, M, R, Niaouli, Cypress, Oregano, Rosemary, Red Thyme, Garlic O, SP

Whooping Cough(protection against): Cinnamon, Clove, Juniper, Ginger, Eucalyptus D, I

BLENDS

Chicken Pox: Blend #6 B, C, N
Chills: Blend #6 B, C
Colds: Blend #6 B, C, D, M, O, SP
Contagious or Infectious Diseases: Blend #6 D, M
Ear Infections: Blend #6 M
Epstein Barr: Blend #6 B, C, D, M, O
Fevers: Blend #6 B, C, D, M, O, P, SP
Flu: Blend #6 B, C, D, M, O, P
Herpes Virus I: Blend #6 B, C, N
Herpes Virus II: Blend #6 B, C, N
Measles: Blend #6 D, M
Valley Fever: Blend #6 B, C, D, M, O, P, SP
Yeast Infection: Blend #6 DO, O, ON

Immune System Testimony

PREVENTIVE—BOBBI CONNER

Since my boys were small, I have relied on Blend #7 whenever they have congestion. In addition to the aromatic properties opening up their respiratory system, the gentle massage soothed and comforted them. They now hand me the oils and throw their feet in my lap.

COLDS AND VIRUSES—ROSALIE WYLIE

I teach handicapped children where I'm exposed to all kinds of things daily. I use Blend #6 daily on my feet and back of neck. This has kept me from all the colds and viruses that I would usually pick up.

EAR INFECTIONS—KARLA CEDARLEAF

My children were constantly having ear infections, colds, and viruses. Blend #6 applied daily before school and before bed kept them from experiencing these problems this year.

Intestinal System

SINGLE OILS

Cleansing: Grapefruit O

Colic: Bergamot, Roman Chamomile, Dill C, D, M, R

Colitis: Dill, Roman Chamomile, Neroli, Rosemary C, E, M, R

Constipation: Black Pepper, Fennel O, Orange, Rosemary, Sweet Marjoram, Bergamot, Peppermint, Lemon E, M, R, SP

Crohn's Disease: Myrrh E, M, R, Neroli E, M, O ,R

Diarrhea: Cinnamon, Roman Chamomile, Cypress, Ginger, Neroli, Nutmeg, Rosemary, Peppermint O Myrrh E

Gas(intestinal): Peppermint, Black Pepper, Cinnamon, Clove ,Dill, Ginger O(spasm) Lemongrass, Sandalwood, Nutmeg ,Sweet Marjoram O Lavender M, N, R

Gastritis: Sandalwood O

Hemorrhoids: Cypress, Geranium, Myrrh, Spikenard, Peppermint B, ON, S, SP

Intestinal(catarrh): Geranium E, SP

Intestinal(ferment): Juniper E, SP

Intestinal Flora(balance): Neroli E, M, SP

Intestinal(infection): Lemon, Nutmeg, Red Thyme, Neroli, Rosemary O Ylang Ylang B, C, M, O

Intestinal(parasites): Bergamot, Eucalyptus, Hyssop, Lemon, Sweet Marjoram, Basil, Red Thyme, Clove, Sweet Thyme, Peppermint C, M, Ô, Lavender C, M

Intestinal(spasms): Basil, Dill, Ginger O

Intestinal(virus): Red Thyme O

Irritable Bowel Syndrome: Cypress, Dill O

Parasites: See intestinal parasites

Spastic Colon: Dill M, O

BLENDS

Colitis/Ulcerative Colitis: Blend #10 C, M

Diarrhea: Blend #10 C, M

Diverticulitis: Blend #7, Blend #10 C, M

Irritable Bowel Syndrome: Blend #10 C, M

Lymphatic System

SINGLE OILS
Cellulite: Cedarwood, Fennel, Grapefruit, Juniper, Lemon, Orange
Gout: Juniper
Lymph Congestion: Cistus, Grapefruit, Orange, Lemon, Juniper, Geranium
Obesity: Grapefruit, Lemon, Patchouli, Fennel
Toxin Removal: Grapefruit, Juniper, Orange, Lemon
Water Retention: Cedarwood, Lemon, Grapefruit

BLENDS
Cellulite: B, M
Swollen Glands: Blend #2 B, M
Weight loss: B, M

Mind System

SINGLE OILS
Acceptance: Pine, Peppermint B, D, I, M
Action: Ginger B, C, M
Addictions: Bergamot, Lavender, Vetiver, Peppermint A, B, D, M, O Vetiver, Peppermint A, B, D, M, R
Agitation: Lavender, Sandalwood A, B, D, M, R
Anger: Roman Chamomile, Rose Bulgarian, Ylang Ylang A, B, D, M, R
Anxiety: Basil, Bergamot, Cedarwood, Geranium, Lavender, Patchouli, Sweet Marjoram, Peppermint, Sandalwood, Ylang Ylang, Juniper, Orange, Roman Chamomile, Ravensara A, B, D, M, R
Apathy: Lemon, Rosemary, Peppermint A, B, D, M, R
Apprehension: Frankincense, Lavender, Sandalwood, Ylang Ylang A, B, D, M, R
Argumentative: Eucalyptus A, B, D, M, R
Awakening: Peppermint A, B, C, D, MO
Attitude(bad): Lemon A, B, C, D, M, O
Balancing Centering: Cistus, Cypress, Eucalyptus A, B, C, D, M, O
Bitter: Lemon A, B, C, D, M, O
Blame and Shame(oneself): Pine D, I, M

Brain Stimulant: Rosemary, Peppermint, Basil D, I, M

Burnout: Lavender, Orange A, B, C, D, M, R

Calm Emotions: Bois de Rose, Sandalwood A, C, D, M, R

Centering: Cistus, Cypress, Eucalyptus D, I, M, R

Circulation: Black Pepper, Rosemary, Basil D

Clarity: Grapefruit, Peppermint, Lemon A, B, C, D, M, R

Cleansing(the mind): Tea Tree A, B, C, D,M, R

Cluttered thoughts: Eucalyptus A, B, C, D, I, M, R

Concentration: Eucalyptus, Peppermint A, B, C, D, I, M, R

Confidence: Grapefruit A, B, C, D, I, M, R

Confusion: Basil, Sweet Marjoram C, M, R, Juniper A, B, C, D, I, M, R

Convalescing: Clary Sage, Lavender, Neroli D, I, M, R

Courage: Cinnamon, Red Thyme O

Creativity(lack of): Fennel O

Creativity(enhancement): Cinnamon O, D

Depletion: Juniper A, B, C, D, I, M, O, R

Depression: Bergamot, Clary Sage, Geranium, Grapefruit, Helichrysum, Peppermint, Neroli, Lavender, Orange, Patchouli, Rose Bulgarian, Rosemary, Sandalwood, Red Thyme, Ylang Ylang A, B, C, D, I, M, R Basil, Clove, Red Thyme A, D, M, R

Despair: Frankincense A, B, C, D, I, M, R

Discontentment: Geranium A, B, C, D, I, M, R

Distrust: Lemon A, B, C, D, I, M, R

Emotional(coldness): Cinnamon O, Cistus A, B, C, D, I, M ,R

Emotional(crisis): Bergamot A, B, C, D, I, M, R

Emotional(refreshing): Peppermint A, B, C, D, I, M, R

Emotional(stability): Neroli, Cedarwood A, B, C, D, I, M, R

Emotional(tension): Spikenard A, B, C, D, I, M, R

Emotional(inner emptiness): Cistus A, B, C, D, I, M, R

Exhaustion: Cinnamon O, D, Lavender, Pine A, B, C ,D, I, M, ON, R

Fear: Basil, Clary Sage, Frankincense, Geranium, Neroli, Lavender, Sweet Marjoram, Ylang Ylang A, B, C, D, I, M, R, Cinnamon O, D

Forgetfulness: Sweet Marjoram, Rosemary A, D, I, M, R

Fretfulness: Roman Chamomile A, B, C, D, I, M ,R

Grief: Frankincense, Rose A, B, C, D, I, M, R

Goals(attainment): Ravensara A, B, C, D, I, M, R

Grounding: Sandalwood, Vetiver A, B, C, D, I, M, R

Heartache: Geranium, Rose A, B, C, D, I, M, R

Helplessness: Peppermint A, B, C ,D, I, M, R

Humor(lack of): Lemon A, B C, D I, M, R

Hysteria: Bergamot, Roman Chamomile, Lavender, Vetiver A, B, C, D, I, M, R

Indecisive: Lemon, Patchouli A, B, C, D, I, M, R

Insecurity: Geranium, Lavender A, B, C, D, I, M, R

Instability: Geranium, Sweet Marjoram A, B, C, D, I, M, R

Irrationality: Lemon A, B, C, D, I, M, R

Irritability: Bergamot, Cedarwood, Geranium, Lavender A, B, C, D, I, M, R

Isolation: Sandalwood A, B, C, D, M, R

Jitters: Lavender A, B, C, D, I, M, R

Lost Inner Child: Lavender A, B, C, D, I, M, R

Low Self Esteem: Geranium A,B,C,D,I,M,R

Meditation: Cedarwood, Cistus, Frankincense, Myrrh A, B, C, D, I, M, R

Memory Loss: Basil, Clove, Rosemary A, B, C, D, I, M, R

Mental(blocks): Lemon A, B, C, D, I, M, R

Mental(clarity): Red Thyme, Peppermint A, B, C, D, I, M, R

Mental(debilitation): Clary Sage A, B, C, D, I, M, R

Mental(fatigue): Basil, Lemon, Rosemary, Peppermint A, B, C, D, I, M, R

Mental(strain): Rosemary A, B, C, D, I, M, R

Mood Swings: Patchouli, Rosemary A, B, C, D, I, M, R

Moodiness: Geranium, Lavender A, B, C, D, I, M, R Cinnamon O, D

Nervousness: Clary Sage, Geranium, Lavender, Roman Chamomile A, B, C, D, I, M, R

Nightmares: Lavender A, B, C, D, I, M, R

Obsessive behavior: Lavender A, B, C, D, I, M, R

Overly excited: Lavender A, B, C, D, I, M, R

Overly quiet: Pine D, I, M, Vetiver A, B, C, M, R

Overly sensitive: Geranium A, B, C, D, I, M, R

Overwhelmed: Dill O, M, R

Overworked: Peppermint A, B, C, D, I, M, O, R

Panic: Lavender A, B, C, D, I, M, R

Post-partum(depression): Jasmine A, B, C, M, ON, R, Clary Sage A, B, C, D, I, M, ON, R

Prayer: Myrrh, Frankincense A, B, C, D, I, M, R

Psychic Abilities: Frankincense A, B, C, D, I, M, R

Punishing Yourself: Pine D, I, M

Regenerating: Peppermint A, B, C, D, I, M, O, R

Relaxant (Nervous System): Cedarwood D, I, Roman Chamomile A, B, C, D, I, M, R

Restlessness: Lavender A, B, C, D, I, M, R

Sadness: Orange, Patchouli, Rosemary, Rose A, B, C, D, I, M, R

Shock: Neroli, Peppermint A, B, C, D, I, M, R

Short Temper: Roman Chamomile, Eucalyptus A, B, C, D, I, M, R

Sluggishness: Rosemary, Tea Tree, Peppermint A, B, C, D, I, M, R

Spirituality: Frankincense, Neroli, Myrrh A, B, C, D, I, M, R

Stimulate Motivation: Black Pepper-D, Fennel O

Stress: Bergamot, Clove, Geranium, Helichrysum, Lemon, Lavender, Patchouli A, B, C, D, M, R

Tension: Cinnamon, Geranium, Helichrysum, Bergamot, Neroli, Lavender A, B, C, D, M, R

Tiredness: Basil, Helichrysum, Tea Tree A, D, M, R

Turmoil: Lemon A, B, C, D, I, M, R

Unable to Adjust: Fennel O

Uncontrollable Sobbing: Cypress A, B, C, D, I, M, R

Understanding: Pine D, I, M

Uplifting: Bergamot, Geranium A, B, C, D, I, M, R

Vibrancy: Peppermint A, B, C, D, I, M, R

Vigor: Tea Tree A, B, C, D, I, M, R

Visualizing(conscious): Cistus A, B, C, D, I, M, R

Vitality: Peppermint A, B, C, D, I, M, R

Warm and Energized Heart: Orange A, B, C, D, I, M, R

Weak Ego: Rosemary A, B, C, D, I, M, R

Weakened State(mentally): Clary Sage, Tea Tree A, B, C, D, I, M, R

Worry: Roman Chamomile, Geranium, Lavender A, B, C, D, I, M, R, Pine A, D, I, M, R

BLENDS

Alcoholism: Blend #2, B, M Blend #10 M, sniff

Anger: Blend #8 B, M, sniff

Anxiety: Blend #8, Blend #9, Blend #10 B, D, M, SN

Clarity: Blend #9 D, M, sniff

Comforting: Blend #8 B, D, M, sniff

Confidence: Blend #9 D, M, sniff

Depression: Blend #7 B, D, M
Grief: Blend #8 B, M, sniff
Hysteria: Blend #9 D, M, sniff
Insecurity: Blend #9 D, M, sniff
Insomnia: Blend #10 A, B, C, D, M, R, sniff
Mental Exhaustion: Blend #9 D, M, sniff
Miscarriage(overcome loss): Blend #10 A, B, C, D, M, R, sniff
Moodiness: Blend #9 D, M, sniff
Parkinson's(emotionally out of control): Blend #10 A, B, C, D, M, R, sniff
Postpartum Blues: Blend #8 B, M, sniff
Replenishing: Blend #9 D, M, sniff
Restlessness: Blend #9 D, M, sniff
Sadness: Blend #8 B, M, sniff
Schizophrenia: Blend #7 A, B, C, D, M, R, sniff
Sedative: Blend #8 B, M, sniff
Stimulating: Blend #9 A, B, C, D, M, sniff
Stress(due to pressure: work or home): Blend #9 A, B, C, D, M, R, sniff
Terminally Ill: Blend #2 A, B, C, M, R
Uplifting: Blend #9 A, B, C, D, M, R, sniff
Worry: Blend #9 A, B, C, D, M, R, sniff

Muscular System

SINGLE OILS

Exercise Preparation: Grapefruit A, B, C, M, ON, R
Inflammation: Cistus, Helichrysum, Lemongrass A, B, C, M, ON, R, S
Leg Cramps: Ginger, Peppermint, Clove, Nutmeg, Eucalyptus C, M, ON, R, S
Muscle(aches): Clary Sage, Grapefruit, Clove, Nutmeg ,Eucalyptus, Ginger A, C, M, ON, R, S
Muscle(fatigue): Black Pepper, Pine, Clove, Nutmeg, Ginger, Eucalyptus, Peppermint A, C, M, ON, R, S
Muscle(pain): Black Pepper, Clary Sage, Grapefruit, Helichrysum, Lemongrass, Nutmeg, Pine, Sweet Marjoram, Ginger, Clove, Rosemary, Peppermint A, C, M, ON, R, S
Muscle(stiffness): Sweet Marjoram, Rosemary, Eucalyptus, Peppermint, Ginger

A, B, C, M, ON, R, S, Clove, Black Pepper, Nutmeg A, M, R

Muscle(tension): Helichrysum, Rosemary, Eucalyptus, Peppermint, Sweet Majoram, Ginger A, B, C, M, ON, R, S, Nutmeg, Clove A, M

Muscle(spasms): Sandalwood, Peppermint A, B, C, M, ON, R, S

Muscle(sprains): Helichrysum, Roman Chamomile, Sweet Marjoram, Cypress, Ginger, Eucalyptus A, B, C, M, ON, R, S, Clove, Nutmeg A, M, R

Muscle(Tension): Helichrysum, Rosemary, Eucalyptus, Peppermint, Sweet Majoram, Ginger A, B, C, M, ON, R, S, Nutmeg, Clove A, M, R

Muscle(strains): Helichrysum, Roman Chamomile, Sweet Marjoram, Cypress, Ginger, Eucalyptus A, B, C, M, ON, R, S, Clove, Nutmeg A, C, M, R

Toning Weak Muscles: Cypress, Lemongrass A, B, C, M, ON, R, S

BLENDS

Fibromyalgia: Blend #4 C, M

Inflammation: Blend #6 B, C, M

Leg Aches: Blend #4 C, M

Lupus (pain): Blend #4 C, M

Pain: Blend #2 B, M

Sprains: Blend #4 B, C, M

Swelling of Sprains: Blend #6 B, C, M

Muscular System Testimony

BRUISING–NANCY JONES

Being a mother of five is a strenuous workout sometimes. One day I fell and bruised my arm. Lorrie made me a massage oil for muscle pain consisting of Sweet Marjoram, Lavender, and Nutmeg. It warmed up my muscles and helped them relax so life could continue normally.

ACHES AND PAINS–LIDDY GEARHEART

Blend #2 has been one of the greatest products that I have ever used. Generally I use Blend #2 for aches and pains, particularly when there is a burning sensations with the aches and pains.

CAT TRAUMA–LIDDY GEARHEART

When my cat was hit by a car, and had to have hip surgery he had a difficult time regarding the use of his leg. At one point the veterinarian said that we should amputate his leg. I held out wanting to give my cat, Ah-He, more time. Several times a day I would rub down his shaved hip with Blend #2, which would enable him to use his leg more. If I forgot to rub him down then he would not try to walk, but as soon as I rubbed him down then he would start using his injured leg. It was quite clear that his hip was sore and that the Blend #2 was relieving the discomfort.

Nervous System

SINGLE OILS

Anorexia: Roman Chamomile, Bergamot, Ginger, Fennel O

Antispasmodic: Bergamot A, B, C, D, I, M, R

Anxiety: Basil, Juniper, Orange, Patchouli, Ravensara, Sweet Marjoram, Lavender

Roman Chamomile: Geranium A, B, C, M, R

Calming: Roman Chamomile, Lavender, Ylang Ylang A, B, C, D, M, R

Convalescence: Neroli, Lavender, Clary Sage A, D, I, M

Convulsions: Clary Sage, Lavender N

Depression: Geranium, Grapefruit, Helichrysum, Neroli, Sandalwood, Sweet Thyme, Basil, Bergamot, Clary Sage, Clove, Lavender A, D, I, M

Epilepsy: Lavender N

Facial Neuralgia: Geranium A, B, C, D, I, M, R

Fatigue: Basil, Clove, Geranium, Helichrysum A, B, C, D, I, M, R

Fear: Neroli,Clary Sage, Frankincense, Geranium, Lavender ,Ylang Ylang, Sweet Marjoram A, B, C, D, I, M, R, Cinnamon O, D. Basil A, D, I, M, R

Frigidity: Bois de Rose, Patchouli, Jasmine, Clary Sage A, B, M, ON, R, Clove, Black Pepper A,M,R

Hang-Over: Clary Sage A, B, C, D, I, M, R

Headache: Basil, Bois de Rose, Roman Chamomile, Clary Sage, Grapefruit, Lemongrass, Lemon, Lavender, Rosemary, Spikenard, Ylang Ylang A, B, C, D, I, M, R

Headache(due to nausea): Bois de Rose A, D, M, R

Herpes(due to stress): Bergamot, Eucalyptus, Tea Tree C, CL, N, ON

High Blood Pressure(due to anxiety): Lavender, Ylang Ylang A, B, C, D, I, M, R

Hyperactivity(due to digestive problems): Roman Chamomile, Peppermint (accident prone, often bumping head), Lavender; use Lavender first if no calming reaction, use Peppermint A, B, C, D, I, M, R

Hypertension: Lemon,Ylang Ylang A, B, C, D, I, M, R

Insomnia: Bergamot, Roman Chamomile, Neroli, Lavender, Orange, Sandalwood, Spikenard, Sweet Marjoram, Vetiver A, B, C, D, I, M, R

Lethargy: Ravensara A, B, C, D, I, M, R

Mental Instability: Sweet Marjoram, Lavender A, B, C, D, I, M, R

Migraines: Clary Sage, Eucalyptus, Lemon, Lavender, Rose Bulgarian, Rosemary A, B, C, D, I, M, R Sweet Marjoram A, C, D, M, O, R, Basil A, D, M, O, R

Nervous(exhaustion): Grapefruit, Patchouli, Sweet Thyme, Vetiver, Sweet Majoram, Bergamot, Peppermint A, B, C, D, M, R

Nervous(indigestion): Spikenard A, B, C, M, R, Roman Chamomile, Dill A, C, M, O, R

Nervous(stimulant): Black Pepper, Red Thyme M, R, Tea Tree A, B, C, D, I, M, R

Nervous(tension): Bois de Rose, Juniper, Neroli, Lavender, Roman Chamomile, Sweet Marjoram, Sweet Thyme, Vetiver, Grapefruit, Patchouli, Helichrysum A, B, C, M, R

Overly Sensitive: Vetiver A, B, C, M, R

Paralysis: Rosemary A, B, C, D, I, M, R

Relaxing: Lavender, Ylang Ylang, Roman Chamomile A, B, C, D, I, M, R

Sharp Stabbing Pain Along Nerves: Helichrysum A, B, C, M, R

Shingles(due to stress): Bergamot, Eucalyptus, Geranium, Rose Bulgarian, Sweet Thyme, Tea Tree A, B, C, N, R

Shock: Neroli, Peppermint, Lavender A, B, C, N, R

Stress: Bois de Rose, Grapefruit, Sweet Marjoram, Sweet Thyme, Juniper, Neroli, Lavender, Roman Chamomile A, B, C, D, I, M, R Helichrysum, Patchouli, Vetiver A, B, C, M, R

Tiredness: Bergamot, Peppermint, Grapefruit, Sweet Thyme, Sweet Marjoram A, B, C, D, I, M, R, Patchouli, Vetiver A, B, C, M, R

Vertigo: Lavender A, B, C, D, I, M, R, Helichrysum A, B, C, M, R

BLENDS

A.D.D.: Blend #5, Blend #7, Blend #10 M

Addictions: Blend #10 Blend #2

Alcoholism: Blend #2, Blend #10 M, sniff

Alzheimer's: Blend #5 D, M

Anxiety and Panic Attack: Blend #7, Blend #9; Blend #10 A, B, C, D, M, R, sniff

Depression: Blend #7, Blend #10(manic) A, B, C, D, M, R, sniff

Dyslexia: Blend #5 M

Exhaustion: Blend #9 D, M, sniff

Headaches: Blend #5 D, M, sniff

High Blood Pressure(stress related): Blend #7,Blend #10 D, M, sniff

Insomnia: Blend #7, Blend #10 A, B, C, D, M, sniff

Irritability: Blend #9 A, B, C, D, M, R, sniff

Nervousness: Blend #9 A, B, C, D, M, R, sniff

Parkinson's(calms emotionally, when feeling out of control): Blend #7, Blend #10 A, B, C, D, M, R, sniff

Schizophrenia: Blend #7 A, B, C, D, M, R, sniff

Seizures(after): Blend #10 A, B, C, D, M, R, sniff

Shingles: Blend #6 C, N, ON

Stress: Blend #7, Blend #9, Blend #10 A, B, C, D, M, R, sniff

Tension: Blend #9 A, B, C, D, M, R, sniff

Tiredness: Blend #9 A, B, C, D, M, R, sniff

Reproductive System

SINGLE OILS

Amenorrhea (lack of period): Clary Sage, Sweet Thyme, Fennel, Rosemary, Nutmeg, Myrrh, Rose Bulgarian A, B, C, Basil, Dill O

Aphrodisiac: Black Pepper, Bois de Rose, Cedarwood, Clary Sage, Clove, Jasmine, Cinnamon, Patchouli, Ylang Ylang, Vetiver, Juniper, Rose Bulgarian, Sandalwood

Balance Hormones: Fennel O

Breast(cancer): Geranium, Lemon A, B, C, R

Breast(engorgement): Geranium, Fennel, Peppermint A, B, C, R

Breast(fibrocystic): Geranium, Lemon, Roman Chamomile A, B, C, M, R

Breast (inflammation): Frankincense A, B, C, M, R

Candida: Myrrh, Sweet Thyme, Bois de Rose, Tea Tree, Neroli, Niaouli, Eucalyptus DO, SP

Childbirth(stimulates contractions): Clary Sage, Clove, Jasmine, Cinnamon,

Peppermint Cedarwood A, M, R

Childbirth(infection): Niaouli B, O, S, SP

Dysmenorrhea(pain associated with menstruation): Clary Sage, Cypress, Geranium, Lemon, Frankincense, Ginger A, M, O

Dysplasia: Niaouli B, S, SP

Edema(pregnancy): Geranium, Lemon A, B, M, R

Endometrosis: Geranium, Clary Sage, Nutmeg, Rose Bulgarian A, B, C, M, O, R

Female problems: Geranium, Clary Sage, Nutmeg ,Rose Bulgarian, Jasmine A, B, C, M, R

Frigidity: Black Pepper, Clary Sage, Jasmine, Lavender, Patchouli, Sandalwood, Bois de Rose, Vetiver, Ylang Ylang A, M, ON, R

Genital Herpes: Ravensara, Rose Bulgarian DO, ON, SP

Genital Irritation: Sweet Marjoram C, M, ON, R

Gonorrhea: Cedarwood, Juniper, Sandalwood, Lemon, Lavender B, C, N, O, S, SP

Grounding(Lower Chakras): Vetiver A, B, C, M, N

Impotence: Black Pepper M,R, Cedarwood M, Clary Sage B, M, R, Clove, Geranium, Ginger, Pine, Cinnamon, Peppermint, Sandalwood O, Ylang Ylang B, C, M, Sweet Thyme SP, Jasmine A, B, M, ON, R

Infertility: Geranium, Rose Bulgaria A, B, C, M, N, ON, R

Jock Itch: Tea Tree, Myrrh B, C, N, ON

Menopause: Roman Chamomile, Clary Sage, Cypress, Fennel, Geranium, Peppermint A, B, C, M, ON, R, Fennel O

Menstrual Problems(cramps): Cedarwood M, Cistus M, R, Eucalyptus C, M, Frankincense A, D, I, M, R, Cinnamon O, Clary Sage B, M, R, Ginger B, M, R, Jasmine, Lavender, Rosemary, Sandalwood, Roman Chamomile, Sweet Marjoram A, B, M, ON, R, Clove A, C, M, O, R

Menstrual Problems(constant period): see dysmenorrhea

Menstrual Problems(pain, scanty): Basil, Lavender, Hyssop, Juniper, Clove, Ginger A, M, R

Menstrual Problems(lack of period): see ammenorrhea

Ovarian Cyst: Cypress, Lemon C, M, O, R

P.M.S.: Bergamot, Clary Sage, Fennel, Frankincense, Geranium, Neroli, Lavender A, B, C, D, I, M, R Vetiver, Peppermint, Ylang Ylang, Nutmeg, Rose Bulgarian A, B, C, M, R, S

Post Partum Blues: Jasmine, Geranium, Rose Bulgarian, Neroli A, B, C, M, R, S

Pregnancy(anxiety): Geranium A, B, M, R, S

Pregnancy(circulation): Lemon A, B, M, R, S

Pregnancy(edema): Geranium, Lemon A, B, M, R, S

Pregnancy(stress): Geranium A, B, M, R, S

Prostate: Sweet Thyme, Jasmine, Sandalwood, Pine, Lemon ,Juniper (see external applications of aromatherapy under ointments, but do apply rectally)

Prostatitis: Sandalwood, Pine, Lemon, Juniper, Roman Chamomile (see internal applications of aromatherapy under suppositories)

Syphilis: Lemon DO, N, ON, SP

Uterine Cancer: Geranium DO, M, N, O, SP

Uterine Hemorrhage: Myrrh DO, SP

Uterus(toning): Geranium, Frankincense, Black Pepper, Clary Sage, Clove, Rose Bulgarian O

Vaginal Discharge: Hyssop, Sweet Thyme, Rosemary DO, O, S, SP

Vaginal Itching: Bergamot, Myrrh, Tea Tree, Lavender, Ravensara B, DO, O, ON, S, SP

Vaginitis: Roman Chamomile, Sweet Thyme, Niaouli, Rose Bulgarian, Tea Tree, Ravensara B, DO, O, SP, Red Thyme O, Lavender, Cedarwood DO, SP

Yeast Infection: Tea Tree, Bois de Rose, Neroli, Niaouli, Myrrh, SweetThyme, Lavender, Ravensara DO, SP

BLENDS

After Child Birth(sitz bath): Blend #7 ON, SB

Aphrodisiac: Blend #8 B, M, SZ

Endometriosis: Blend #3 M, SP

Female Douche: Blend #6 DO

Female Problems: Blend #3, Blend #10 A, B, C, D, DO, M, R, sniff

Frigidity: Blend #8 B, M, sniff

Hot Flashes: Blend #3 B, D, M, SZ, sniff

Impotence: Blend #8 M, sniff

Infertility: Blend #3 M

Menopause: Blend #3, Blend #10 A, B, C, M, R, sniff

Menstrual Cramps: Blend #3, Blend #8 A, B, C, D, M, R, sniff

Miscarriage: Blend #7 A, B, C, D, M, R, sniff

P.M.S.: Blend #3, Blend #7, Blend #10 A, B, C, D, M, R, sniff

Postpartum Blues: Blend #7, Blend #8 A, B, C, D, M, R, sniff

Yeast Infections: Blend #6 DO, ON, SP

Reproductive System Testimony

UTERINE FIBROID CYST—MARY FUGITT

I was diagnosed with fibroid cysts three years ago. My symptoms included heavy monthly cycles, and two periods that lasted for 48 days. My doctor said it was probably fibroids and ordered an ultra sound to confirm. Another appointment was set for four weeks later to recheck growth. In the mean time, I began an herbal regime that consisted of Special Formula, FC with Dong Quai, vitamin E, vitamin A & D, and Pau D' Arco. I also used an essential oil blend created by Lorrie Hargis consisting of Roman Chamomile, Lemon, and Geranium. I rubbed the blend on my abdomen in the morning and at night before I went to bed. In four weeks when the ultra sound was performed, the fibroids had shrunk to the size of a fingertip. My monthly cycle had returned to normal. This took a total of three months.

HOT FLASHES—KAY LUBECKE

I mixed 7 drops of Blend #3 in 1 T. of massage oil. At bedtime, I apply several drops to my abdomen and rub it until it is almost all absorbed. Since doing this, I am experiencing far fewer hot flashes at night and sleeping much better.

P.M.S.—BOBBI CONNER

I reach for Blend #3 whenever I feel a little irritable, whether its premenstrual or just everyday stress. Just rubbing it into my feet calms me almost immediately.

Respiratory System

SINGLE OILS

Air Disinfectant: Eucalyptus, Pine, Lemon D, I

Antimicrobial: Myrrh, Lemon B, I, M, R, S

Antiseptic: Clove, Pine, Lemon D, I

Asthma: Roman Chamomile, Frankincense, Helichrysum, Hyssop, Lemon, Lavender, Pine, Sweet Thyme, Sweet Marjoram, Peppermint A, B, C, M, R

Bronchitis: Basil, Cedarwood, Frankincense, Helichrysum, Hyssop, Myrrh,

Peppermint, Lemon, Niaouli, Pine, Ravensara, Sweet Marjoram, Sweet Thyme A, D, I, M, SP, Sandalwood A, M, S, P, Dill, Fennel, Red Thyme O

Catarrh(mucous): see congestion

Colds: Rosemary, Tea Tree, Bergamot, Sweet Thyme, Peppermint, Helichrysum, Lemon, Orange A, B, C, D, I, M, O, ON, R, SP Clove, Cinnamon, Red Thyme A, D, M, O, R, Myrrh, Frankincense, Bois de Rose A, B, C, D, I, M, R, SP

Congestion: Cedarwood, Lavender, Frankincense C, M, R, Niaouli, Eucalyptus, Peppermint A, B, C, D, I, M, O, ON, SP, Black Pepper D, M, R

Cough: Cedarwood C, M, Cypress O, Frankincense A, D, I, M, R, SP, Ginger (moist) B, C, I, M, Helichrysum O, Jasmine A, B, C, I, M, ON, R, Lavender B, D, M, Pine D, I, M, Sweet Thyme D, I, M, SP

Earache: Lavender, Rosemary, Sweet Thyme, Eucalyptus, Helichrysum; Garlic (herbal infused oil) see recipe in Immune System.

Expectorant: Sweet Marjoram, Fennel, Cypress O, Eucalyptus, Peppermint A, B, C, D, I, M, O, ON, R, SP, Frankincense, Jasmine, Myrrh, Sandalwood B, C, I, M, R, S, P, Red Thyme, Basil M, O, R, Clove, Cedarwood, Black Pepper D, M, R, Pine D, I

Hay Fever: Roman Chamomile D, I, M, O, Hyssop O

Influenza(protection against): Hyssop, Red Thyme O, Sweet Thyme, Rosemary, Lemon, Niaouli, Peppermint D, I, M, O, R Pine D, I, Lavender D, I, M, R

Influenza(recovery): Cypress, Eucalyptus I, O, Fennel O

Laryngitis: Frankincense, Jasmine, Sandalwood, Rose Bulgarian G, M

Pneumonia: Lemon, Niaouli, Eucalyptus A, B, C, D, I, M, R

Rhythmic Breathing: Ylang Ylang, Frankincense A, B, C, D, I, M, R

Sinus: Basil, Eucalyptus, Niaouli, Ravensara, Rosemary, Sandalwood, Red Thyme, Peppermint A, C, D, I, M, R

Throat Infections: Clary Sage, Eucalyptus, Geranium, Myrrh, Niaouli (strep), Sandalwood, Sweet Thyme, Rose Bulgarian, Tea Tree C, D, G, I, M, R

Tonsillitis: Sweet Thyme, Tea Tree, Sandalwood, Rose Bulgarian, Eucalyptus C, D, G, I, M, R

Tuberculosis: Hyssop, Niaouli, Ravensara, Peppermint, Clove, Eucalyptus C, D, I, M, R, SP

Whooping Cough: Basil, Clary Sage, Cypress, Eucalyptus, Niaouli, Ravensara, Sweet Thyme, Cistus C, D, I, M, R, SP

BLENDS

Asthma: Blend #10(calming) C, M, ON
Bronchitis: Blend #1 D, I, M, O
Cough: Blend #1, Blend #6 with Clary Sage D, I, M, O
Decongestant: Blend #1 D, I, M, O
Laryngitis: Blend #1 D, G, I, M, O
Lung: Blend #1 D, I, M, O
Pneumonia: Blend #1 D, I, M, O
Sinus Congestion: Blend #1 D, I, M, O
Sore Throat: Blend #1 D, G, I, M, O
Strep Throat: Blend #1, Niaouli D, G, I, M, O
Tonsillitis: Blend #1 D, G, I, M, O

Respiratory System Testimony
COUGH–KAY LUBECKE

Don is finally over the cough that followed the severe sinus infection lots of people are experiencing here in Phoenix. After 5 weeks of coughing, we put the following in a diffuser: 10 drops Pine, 10 drops Clove, 5 drops Lemon. He sat in front of the diffuser 10 minutes, three times a day. The coughing was gone in 2 days!

I also use the same formula every time I get a scratchy throat which prevents it from becoming a full-blown infection.

Skeletal System

SINGLE OILS

Arthritis: Black Pepper, Cypress, Ginger, Helichrysum, Juniper, Myrrh, Lemon,Grapefruit Lavender, Patchouli, Red Thyme, Sweet Thyme, Vetiver, Roman Chamomile
Backache: Spikenard, Clove, Peppermint, Rosemary, Helichrysum
Dental Infection: Clove, Lemon,Tea Tree
Dull Aches: Roman Chamomile
General Pain Killer: Clove, Peppermint, Helichrysum
Osteoporosis: Lavender
Rheumatism: Black Pepper, Roman Chamomile, Cypress, Eucalyptus, Ginger, Juniper, Lemon, Lavender, Niaouli, Pine, Red Thyme, Sweet Thyme

Rheumatoid Arthritis: see Rheumatism
Toothache: Black Pepper, Roman Chamomile, Clove, Nutmeg, Cinnamon, Peppermint
Teething: Roman Chamomile

BLENDS
Arthritis: Blend #2, Blend #4
Back(bad disks): Blend #4
Backache: Blend #4
Broken Bones: Blend #4
Carpal Tunnel Syndrome: Blend #4
Fractured Bones: Blend #4
Lupus(pain): Blend #4
Rheumatism: Blend #2

Skeletal System Testimonies
UPPER JAW SURGERY—MRS CINDI WHITESIDE

A carticotomy surgery (upper jawbone manipulation) has a post-surgery outcome of moderate discomfort, tenderness, bruising in various facial areas, sinus sensitivity, and swelling.

A pre-surgery treatment of Zinc, vitamin E, vitamin C, and Arnica enhanced my surgery success, with Arnica as an immediate post-surgery therapy. However, my swelling, tenderness, and sinus sensitivity was minimized by lymphatic massage and gentle pressure point stimulation with the use of an aromatherapy oil blend. This soothing combination of Roman Chamomile, Peppermint, and Lemon was so soothing that it encouraged me to massage all facial and neck areas one to three times a day, stimulating circulation and penetration of oils. This blend limited the swelling and tenderness, stimulated my circulation and created a calming effect. I also used a few drops in my bath water.

I will be applying this blend again after my lower jaw surgery. As an adult, enduring orthodontic and corrective jaw surgery I recommend not only this blend, but other blends such as Blend #10 for calming and healing effects.

ANKLE—SARAH JONES

I have been a competitive soccer player for seven years. My four siblings play also. As with any sport, in soccer you can get injured. I have seen broken bones, bad sprains, and concussions. You name it; I have seen it. A few months ago I was tackled in a collegiate soccer game. My ankle snapped backwards extremely hard. I knew right way that it was bad. My mother immediately took me to Lorrie's and she made a blend consisting of Sweet Marjoram, Roman Chamomile, and Cypress. I did not experience any bruising or noticeable swelling.

I went to the emergency room to get x-rays. The doctor said I had experienced a stress fracture, but I needed a second opinion. The second opinion said that I was fine. It did not look as if any thing was wrong. I began physical therapy on my "bad sprain." The constant pain made the injury become numb.

After two weeks of therapy I was released. I began to practice with my ankle taped. Within two days, I knew that it was not healed. I went to a sports doctor this time, and he said it was a stress fracture, and I needed to allow the ankle time to heal. There was no swelling or bruising of the ankle with the use of this blend.

Skin and Hair Systems

SINGLE OILS

Abscesses: Roman Chamomile, Frankincense, Lavender, Red Thyme, Sweet Thyme C, L, N, ON

Acne: Cedarwood, Eucalyptus, Frankincense, Grapefruit, Peppermint, Lemongrass, Lavender, Patchouli, Rosemary, Sandalwood, Sweet Thyme, Tea Tree, Vetiver, Ylang Ylang, Jasmine C, CL, FA

Acne(Rosacea): Lavender C, CL, FA

Anti-aging: Lavender C, CL, FA, M, ON

Antifungal: Cedarwood, Tea Tree, Patchouli, Myrrh, Lemongrass Geranium, Rosemary B, C, CL, M, ON, S

Antiseptic: Lavender, Orange, Rose Bulgarian, Sweet Thyme, Tea Tree, Niaouli B, C, D, I, N, S, Cinnamon, Clove C, D, I

Athlete's Foot: Lemongrass, Myrrh, Sweet Thyme, Tea Tree, Peppermint,

Niaouli B, C, CL, M, N, ON

Bleeding(stop): Lemon C, N

Blemishes: Eucalyptus, Rosemary, Lavender, Tea Tree, Geranium, Patchouli C, CL, FA, N

Blonde Hair Highlights: Roman Chamomile-Shampoo, spritzer

Boils: Roman Chamomile, Lavender, Patchouli, Red Thyme, Sweet Thyme C, CL, ON

Brittle Nails: Lemon N

Bruises: Fennel, Hyssop, Helichrysum, Peppermint, Rosemary C, CL, M, ON

Brunette Hair (Red) Highlights: Rosemary shampoo, spritzer

Burns: Lavender, Niaouli, Sweet Marjoram C, CL, N, ON

Calluses: Cistus C, CL, N, ON

Canker Sores: Peppermint, Tea Tree, Lavender, Bergamot C, CL, N, ON

Chicken Pox: Eucalyptus, Ravensara, Niaouli, Tea Tree, Lavender, Bergamot, Geranium C, CL, N, ON

Corns: Lemon C, CL, N, ON

Cuts and Wounds: Cedarwood, Roman Chamomile, Frankincense, Juniper, Hyssop, Myrrh, Lemon C, ON, Lavender, Niaouli, Sweet Thyme, Tea Tree, Eucalyptus C, N, ON

Dandruff: Eucalyptus, Tea Tree, Juniper N, shampoo

Deodorant: Eucalyptus, Lemongrass, Tea Tree, Vetiver, Sandalwood B, C, M, ON

Eczema: Lavender, Cistus, Hyssop, Myrrh, Rose Bulgarian, Sweet Thyme B, C, ON

Eczema(weeping): Juniper, Myrrh B, C, ON

Feet(tender): Lemon M, ON

Freckles: Lemon M,ON

Frostbite: Geranium M, N, ON

Gingivitis: Cinnamon, Lemon oral rinse

Gums(receding): Myrrh, Lemon C, G, oral rinse

Gums(tonic): Lemon, Orange C,G, oral rinse

Hair Care: Sandalwood, Rosemary, Roman Chamomile M, shampoo

Herpes(Simplex I): Eucalyptus, Ravensara, Tea Tree, Geranium, Lavender C, CL, N, ON

Herpes(Genital Simplex II): Juniper Lavender Sandalwood N, ON

Herpes(Zoster shingles): Geranium, Neroli, Lemon, Lemongrass, Peppermint, Eucalyptus, Ravensara, Tea Tree, Sweet Thyme, Rose Bulgarian C, CL, N, ON

Insect Bites: Basil, Lemon, Lavender, Patchouli, Sweet Thyme, Tea Tree, Peppermint C, CL, M, ON, spritzer

Insect Repellent: Cedarwood, Eucalyptus, Geranium, Lemongrass, Tea Tree, Peppermint M, ON, spritzer

Jock Itch: Myrrh, Tea Tree N, mix 2 drops of essential oils with 1T. cornstarch or powder. Sprinkle on affected area

Lice: Lemongrass, Geranium M, ON, spritzer

Measles: Eucalyptus, Ravensara, Cistus, Cypress B, C, M, N, S

Mouth Ulcers: Myrrh, Lemon, Orange, Tea Tree N, ON, oral rinse

Nose Bleed: Lemon, put Lemon essential oil directly on cotton ball, and insert in nostril.

Oily Hair: Clary Sage shampoo

Psoriasis: Roman Chamomile, Cistus, Lavender, Spikenard, Sweet Thyme B, C, N, ON

Pyorrhea: Fennel oral rinse

Ringworm: Myrrh, Patchouli, Tea Tree B, C, M, ON

Scabies: Lemongrass, C, ON

Scarlet Fever: Eucalyptus B, C, M, N, ON

Scars: Clary Sage, Frankincense, Geranium, Myrrh, Neroli, Lavender, Niaouli, Patchouli, Sandalwood B, C, CL, M, N, ON, Red Thyme, Cedarwood, Hyssop C, M, ON

Shingles: Eucalyptus, Ravensara, Rose Bulgarian, Sweet Thyme, Tea Tree C, CL, N, ON

Shingles (Herpes Zoster): see Herpes

Skin(dry/oily combination): Bois de Rose, Geranium C, CL, FA, I, M

Skin(dry, sensitive skin): Jasmine, Myrrh, Lavender Patchouli, Clary Sage, Cistus, Sandalwood, Spikenard, Roman Chamomile, RoseBulgarian C, FA, I, M

Skin(oily): Basil, Bergamot, Fennel, Geranium, Grapefruit, Lemon, Rosemary, Vetiver, Roman Chamomile, Clary Sage, Cistus, Cedarwood C, CL, FA

Skin(mature): Jasmine, Spikenard B, C, CL, I, M, N, ON

Skin(open pores): Lemongrass, Lavender, Patchouli B, C, CL, N

Skin(regenerate cells and tissue): Patchouli, Geranium, Sandalwood B, C, CL, M, N, ON

Skin(toning): Grapefruit, Vetiver, Geranium, Neroli, Jasmine B, C, CL, M, N, ON

Skin(ulcers): Clary Sage, Eucalyptus, Geranium, Lavender, Niaouli B, C, CL, M, N, ON

Skin Infections: Sandalwood, Tea Tree, Lavender B, C, CL, N, ON, S

Sores: Patchouli, Tea Tree C, N, ON

Sores(tongue and mucous membranes): Geranium oral rinse

Stretch Marks: Geranium, Jasmine, Neroli, Lavender, Vetiver M, ON

Sunburn: Roman Chamomile, Eucalyptus, Lavender, Peppermint put 5 drops of any one of these essential oils in 1T. Aloe vera gel. Apply to sunburned area.

Swelling: Peppermint B, M, N, ON, S

Thrush: Myrrh N, oral rinse

Toothache: Nutmeg, Clove, Cinnamon, Roman Chamomile, Peppermint, Black Pepper; put 2 drops of any one of these essential oils in 1 1/2 t. of Aloe vera gel. Apply to affected area.

Warts: Lemon N, ON

Wounds: Hyssop, Juniper, Lavender, Lemon, Myrrh, Niaouli, Sweet Thyme, Tea Tree, Cedarwood, Frankincense, Roman Chamomile C, ON

Wrinkles: Bois de Rose, Clary Sage, Lemon C, CL, FA, M, ON

BLENDS

Balancing: Blend #9 C, FA, M

Cold Sores: Blend #6 C, CL, M, N, ON

Cuts: Blend #6 C, M, N, ON

Diaper Rash: Blend #6 C, M, N, ON

Dry Skin: Blend #8 C, FA, I, M, N, ON

Oily Skin: Blend #9 C, CL, FA

Perfume: Blend #8 N

Toning: Blend #9 C, CL, FA

Wounds: C, N, ON

Skin and Hair System Testimony

COSMETIC EYE SURGERY—KALLY ELTON

In 1996 my husband and I attended an Aromatherapy weekend workshop at a resort and health spa, located in the mountains of West Virginia. It was an exciting opportunity for us to learn about the many different types of essential oils and their origins. The weekend proved to be a fascinating and educational experience, but it wasn't until I decided to have a blepharoplasty the next year that I truly experienced the healing effects of nature's most fragrant substances.

After my surgery I returned home with all kinds of lotions and potions prescribed by my plastic surgeon to apply regularly to my fresh eyelid incisions. I was asked to return four days later to have the stitches removed. Even though I didn't feel any real pain from the incisions, I felt a tremendous itching sensation. I had discussed the possibilities of using Lavender as an aid in my healing process with my Aromatherapy instructor prior to my surgery. Since I was not getting the relief from the medicine prescribed by my doctor I decided to try it.

It was like an instant refreshing miracle. I can honestly describe my first application of Lavendula as immediate relief. The itching was gone and it had quite a calming effect. My skin absorbed the Lavender like a sponge absorbs water. I could actually feel my skin healing with each application. I continued my applications twice daily and within a few days you would not believe that I had just had surgery.

When I returned to have my stitches removed my doctor could not believe his eyes. He was surprised and puzzled with my progress. He expected to see some swelling and bruising to my eyes. Instead he described my healing progress of four days similar to a patient after a couple weeks of healing. I continued the Lavender applications after the stitches were removed and saw him again in two weeks. Again his reaction was the same, concerning my rapid healing and non-discernible scarring.

I can truly attribute the successful outcome of my blepharoplasty to my great plastic surgeon and nature's incredible essential oil, Lavender.

MOSQUITO BITES–TERRI HICKS

Texans are first to brag about how big everything is here in God's Country. Well, unfortunately, that includes mosquitoes, flies, and other no-see-ums. The summer of 1998 we experienced an excessive heat wave. Along with the heat came the problem of insects, in particular, the Tiger Mosquito, which is small, but very aggressive. All through spring and early summer we faithfully used Bug Bite Blend and suffered no bites!

When we finished our bottle of Bug Bite Blend, I did not refill it immediately. Within a few days we all had suffered numerous bites, mostly on our legs. Not only were we bothered by the itching, but the wounds were scarring our skin. I immediately purchased more of the blend, and found not only did the bites stop, but also the wounds began to heal quickly without scarring.

We have tried many over the counter insect repellents with all those nasty toxins. I hate to use them on my children, but did so for years because the mosquitoes are such a problem. Bug Bite Blend is a safe product with better results.

BUG BITE BLEND RECIPE
  10 drops Lavender
  10 drops Eucalyptus
  20 drops Sweet Thyme
  2oz. carrier oil

Mix essential oils in 2 oz. bottle. Add carrier oil and rub the bottle back and forth between your hands to blend the oils. Apply to areas where bugs may bite.

Urinary System

SINGLE OILS

Bedwetting: Rosemary O

Bladder Infection: Roman Chamomile, Frankincense, Juniper, Pine, Eucalyptus, Niaouli, Sweet Marjoram, Clove, Sandalwood O Cedarwood, Cistus, Frankincense C, M

Disinfectant Urinary Tract: Bergamot O

Edema: Cypress, Fennel, Orange, Rosemary, Grapefruit, Lemon, Dill, Juniper O Lavender, Patchouli, Cedarwood C, M, R

Gout: Fennel, Juniper O

Kidney Infection: Bergamot, Roman Chamomile, Red Thyme, Sweet Thyme, Sandalwood O

Kidney Stones(dissolve): Fennel, Lemon O

Prostatitis: Pine, Sandalwood, Lemon, Roman Chamomile, Juniper O, SP, Jasmine ON, SP

Urethra(infection): Niaouli O

BLADDER INFECTION RECIPE(INTERNAL USE)
   3 drops Fennel essential oil
   8 drops Lemon essential oil
   4 drops Geranium essential oil
   2 t. Solubol™
   2 t. water

Squeeze Solubol™ into glass, stir in essential oils and water. Drink 15 drops three times daily.

BLENDS
   Diuretic: Blend #2
   Gout: Blend #2
   Water Retention: Blend #2

Section 7

Reflexology Charts

Circulatory System

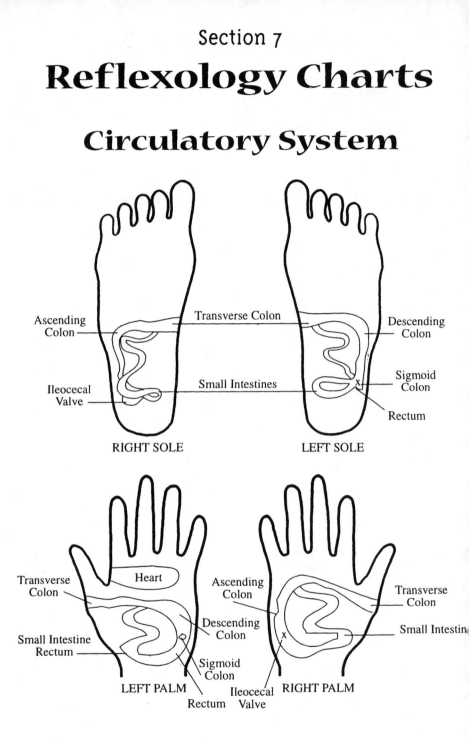

Digestive System

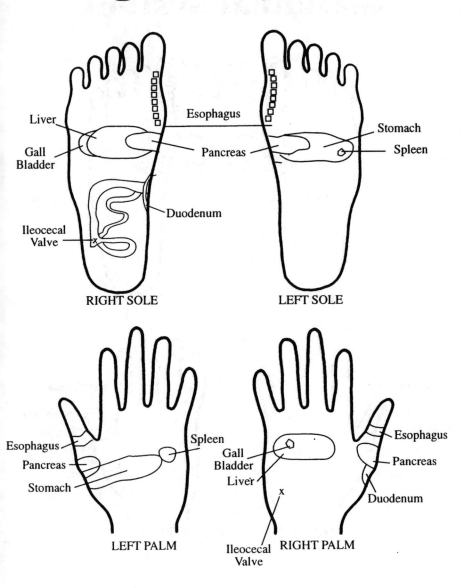

Glandular System

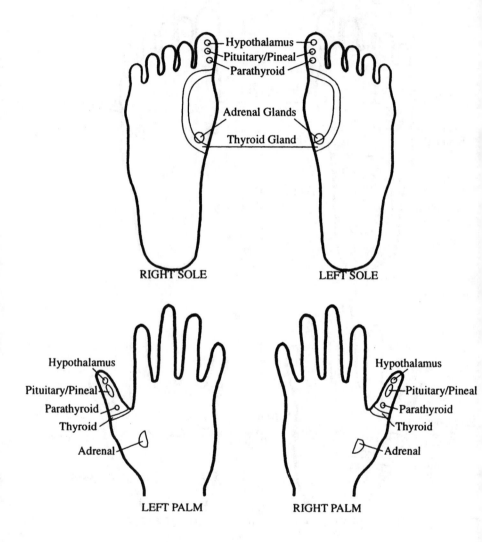

Hypothalamus
Pituitary/Pineal
Parathyroid

Adrenal Glands
Thyroid Gland

RIGHT SOLE   LEFT SOLE

Hypothalamus
Pituitary/Pineal
Parathyroid
Thyroid
Adrenal

Hypothalamus
Pituitary/Pineal
Parathyroid
Thyroid
Adrenal

LEFT PALM   RIGHT PALM

Immune System

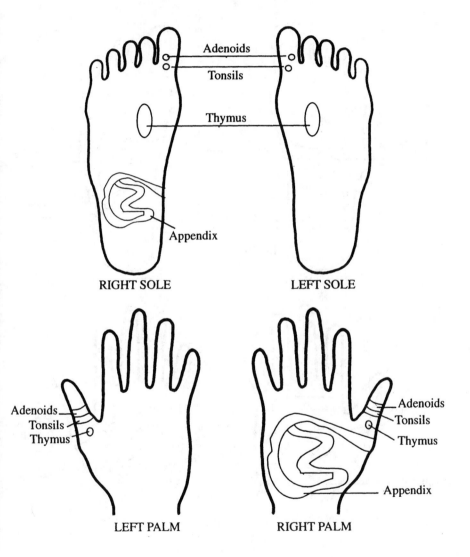

RIGHT SOLE   LEFT SOLE

LEFT PALM   RIGHT PALM

Intestinal System

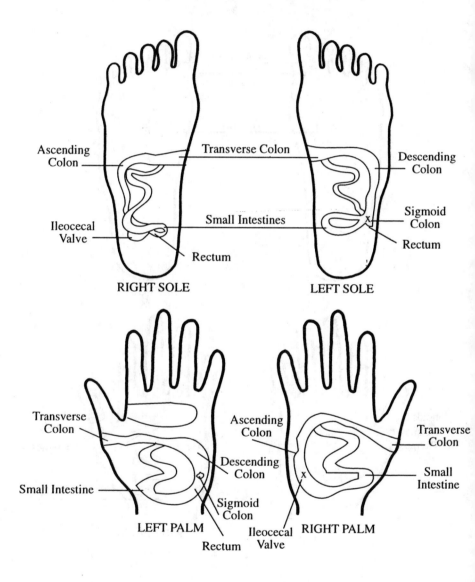

Ascending Colon

Transverse Colon

Descending Colon

Ileocecal Valve

Small Intestines

Sigmoid Colon

Rectum

Rectum

RIGHT SOLE

LEFT SOLE

Transverse Colon

Ascending Colon

Transverse Colon

Descending Colon

Small Intestine

Small Intestine

Sigmoid Colon

LEFT PALM

Ileocecal Valve

RIGHT PALM

Rectum

Lymphatic System

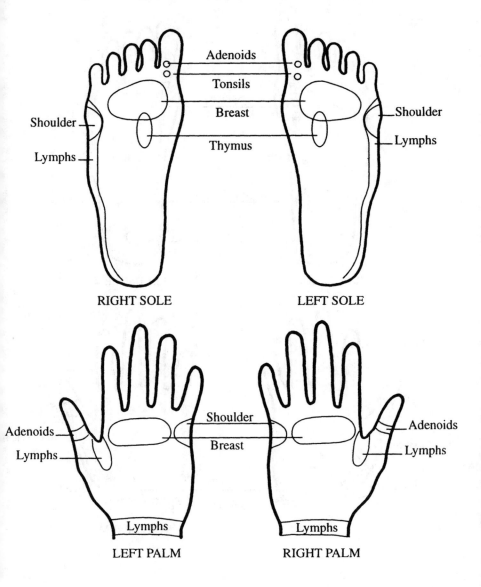

Adenoids
Tonsils
Breast
Thymus

Shoulder
Lymphs

Shoulder
Lymphs

RIGHT SOLE   LEFT SOLE

Shoulder
Breast

Adenoids
Lymphs

Adenoids
Lymphs

Lymphs   Lymphs

LEFT PALM   RIGHT PALM

Muscle System

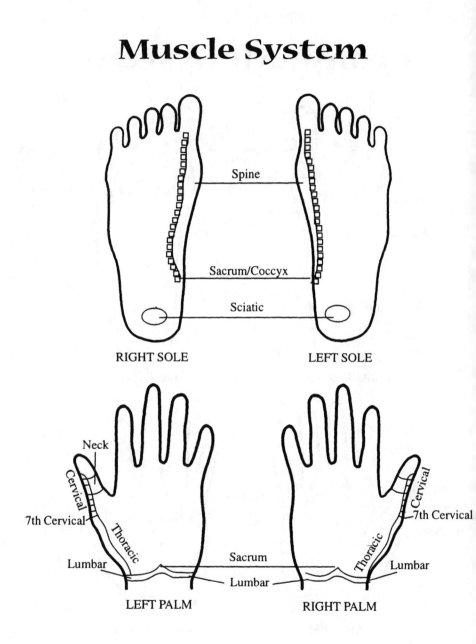

Nervous System

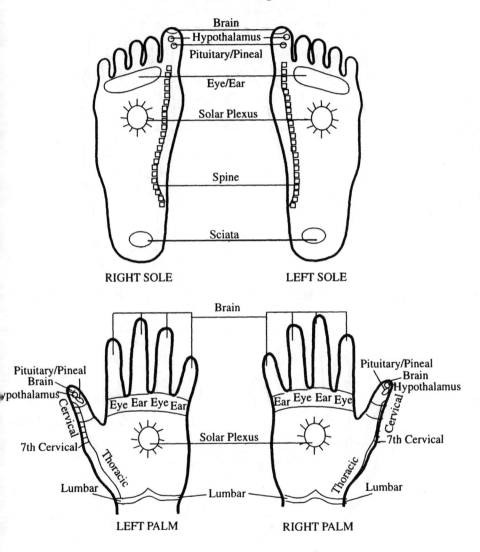

Respiratory System

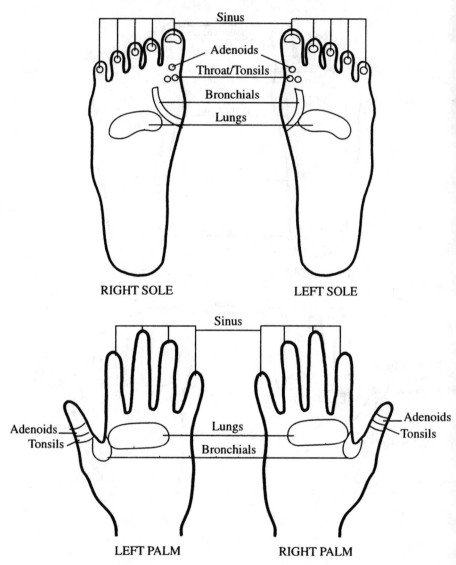

Skeletal System

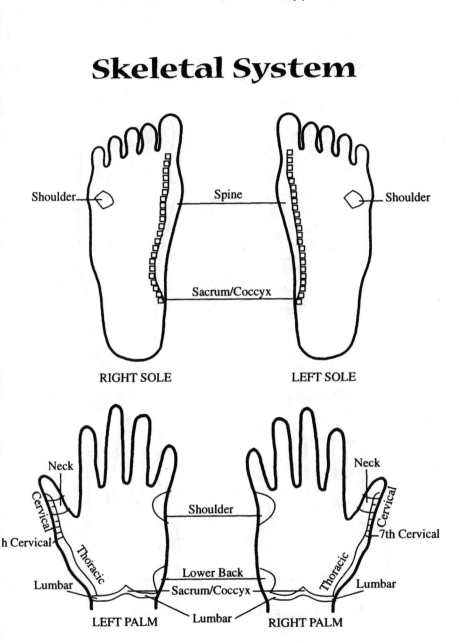

Urinary System

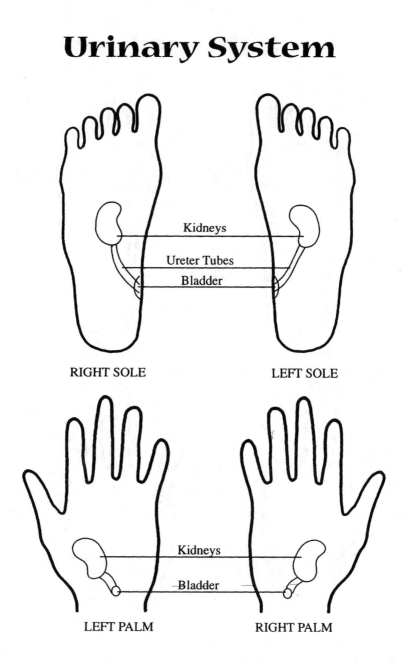

RIGHT SOLE   LEFT SOLE

LEFT PALM   RIGHT PALM

Reproductive System

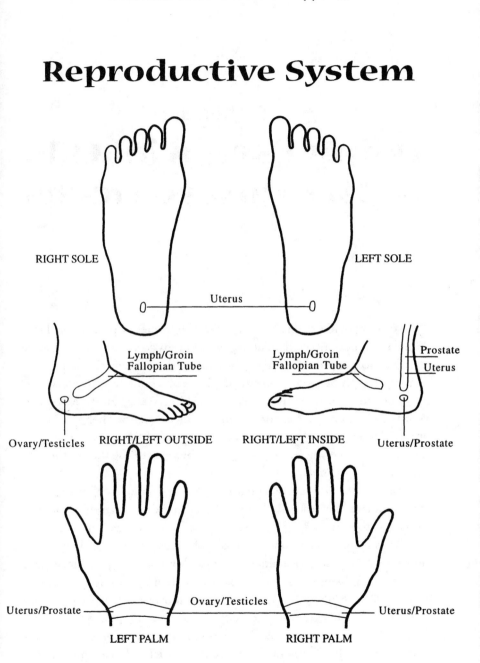

Section 8

Using Essential Oils with Chinese Herbs

I have always had excellent results using the Chinese Constitutional formulas with essential oils. The suggested herbs go directly to the source of imbalance, and the essential oils enhance this synergistic action.

First of all, it helps to understand a little bit about constitutional typing. Chinese philosophy has 5 elements: Fire, Water, Earth, Metal and Wood. Each element has corresponding meridians or energy channels often referred to in Western science as organs of the body. This makes it very easy to see where your imbalances are and to use the appropriate constitutional formula.

Each element also has two polarities, Yin and Yang, with corresponding meridians for each polarity. These meridians can become too stressed—too much Yang, or too weakened—too much Yin.

A stressed person is one who is ambitious, driven, goal oriented, always pushes against deadlines, worries about satisfying superiors and those working beneath them, recovers quickly from illness and trauma, eats too fast, drinks too much and sleeps too little. If a person is too stressed and/or hyperactive, they suffer from too much Yang.

A weakened person is one who recovers slowly from illness and trauma, habitually allows others to take on the burdens of deadlines and has difficulty setting and achiving goals and satisfying the demands of impatient individuals. Frequently seeks out various health professionals, feels larthargic and exhausted. If a person is too weakened and/or hypoactive, they suffer from too much Yin.

Elements

Fire

Corresponding meridians or energy channels: heart (Yin), small intestines (Yang), triple burner (Yang), pericardium (Yin). *The Web Has No Weaver* by Ted J. Kaptchuk is a good source of information on Chinese medicine.

FIRE STRESSED

Inflammation, hypertension, hot tempered, workaholic, does not want to stop and continues on until they can no longer go, sexual impotence, anxiety, insomnia, seized with fright, heart palpitations, pain and distress in the chest. The fire stressed individual does not want to deal with his emotions.

Essential oils help the Fire Stressed individual with these benefits:
Stimulates the circulation and digestion.
Strengthens and brings balance to the emotions.
Increases sexual desire.
Supports the nervous system.

Fire Stressed Single Essential Oils:
Rose, Lavender, Clary Sage, Geranium, Grapefruit, Orange, Lemon, Neroli, Bergamot, Roman Chamomile, and Sweet Marjoram A, B, C, D, M, ON, R (please refer to the codes in the front of the chapter Systems of the Body and Ailments), Ylang-Ylang A, B, C, M, ON, R

Fire Stressed Blends:
Blend #8, Ylang Ylang, Rose, Sandalwood, and Jasmine B, M, ON, R
Blend #10, Bergamot, Roman Chamomile, Geranium, Rose, and Neroli A, B, C, D, M, R

Blend #7, Roman Chamomile, Lavender, Geranium, Mandarin A, B, C, D, M, R.

An shen is the chinese constitutional herbal formula that compliments the essential oils for fire stressed An Shen.

FIRE WEAKENED

Insomnia, dry skin, depression, anemia, poor digestion, sexual weakness, poor memory, mental confusion, heart palpitations and minor chest pains, broken heart, burn out and no passion for their loved ones and/or jobs.

Essential oils help the Fire Weakened individual with these benefits:
Improves digestion.
Increases strength.
Overcomes chronic nervous disorders.
Clears confused thinking and mental frustration.
Relieves depression.

Fire Weakened Single Essential Oils:
Rosemary, Ylang Ylang, Rose, Cedarwood, Cypress, Lemon, Basil, Orange, Bergamot, Grapefruit A, B, C, D, M, R, Ginger, Black Pepper, Nutmeg, Vetiver, Spikenard, Myrrh A, M, R.

Fire Weakened Blends
Blend #5 Rosemary, Basil, Lavender, Grapefruit A, B, C, D, M, R

RECIPE TO STRENGTHEN FIRE WEAKENED INDIVIDUALS:
8 drops Black Pepper essential oil
16 drops Ylang Ylang essential oil
8 drops Orange essential oil
1 oz. massage oil or Solubol™

Place essential oils in 1 oz. bottle and add massage oil/Solubol™. Roll the bottle back and forth between your hands to blend the oils. Pour a few drops into your hand. Hold the oil a few seconds to warm it before applying it to the weakened area. Massage on chest, back, and corresponding reflex points on the feet and hands, twice daily. You could also apply to acupressure points P6, P7.

Yang Xin is the Chinese Constitutional Herbal formula that compliments the essential oils for Fire Weakened.

Earth

Corresponding meridians and energy channels: stomach (Yang), spleen (Yin), and pancreas (Yin).

EARTH STRESSED

Overprotective, slow digestion and intestinal tract, gas, bloating, diahrrea headaches, sluggish energy, too much moisture, foul smelling breath and tired after eating.

Essential oils help the Earth Stressed individual with these benefits:
Relieves gas, bloating, nausea, sleepiness that arises after eating and sluggish digestion.
Reduces mucous congestion.
Balances appetite and weight.

Earth Stressed Single Essential Oils:
Ginger, Orange, Peppermint, Fennel, Hyssop, Sweet Marjoram, Basil, Black Pepper, Juniper A, C, M, O, R.

RECIPE TO RELIEVE GAS FOR EARTH STRESSED INDIVIDUALS:
    10 drops Ginger essential oil
    10 drops Peppermint essential oil
    10 drops Orange essential oil
    1 oz. massage oil or Solubol™

Place essential oils in 1 oz. bottle and add massage oil/Solubol™. Roll the bottle back and forth between your hands to blend the oils. Pour a few drops into your hand. Hold the oil a few seconds to warm it before applying it to the stressed area. Massage corresponding reflex points on feet and hands, you could also apply to acupressure point ST 3.

Xiao Dao is the Chinese Constitutional·Herbal formula that complements the essential oils for Earth Stressed.

EARTH WEAKENED
Cold, hiatal hernia, stomach cramps, prolapsed internal organs (hemorrhoids), diarrhea, chills in arms and legs, fatigue, menstrual cramps, leg cramps, dry and sallow skin, flu, depression, colitis, anorexia, ulcers, emotionally unable to "stomach much", cannot handle a lot of emotion or information. The center of our body is the stomach region. Not only do we digest our food there, we digest our feelings and thoughts, and form opinions in this area.

Essential oils help the earth weakened individual with these benefits:
Improves digestion and assimilation of food.
Strengthens weak muscles.
Warms the internal organs.
Relieves inflammation and infection of the intestines.

Earth Weakened Single Essential Oils:
Roman Chamomile, Ginger, Dill, Orange, Neroli, Lemon, Bergamot, Clove, Nutmeg A, B, C, M, O, R, Black Pepper, Hyssop, Lemongrass O Lavender A, B, C, D, M, R.

RECIPE FOR HIATAL HERNIA AND INDIGESTION FOR EARTH WEAKENED INDIVIDUALS:
9 drops Roman Chamomile essential oil
3 drops Dill essential oil
6 drops Mandarin essential oil
12 drops Lavender essential oil
1 oz massage oil or Solubol™

Place essential oils in 1 oz. bottle and add massage oil/Solubol™. Roll the bottle back and forth between your hands to blend the oils. Pour a few drops into your hand. Hold the oil a few seconds to warm it before applying it to the weakened area. Massage on stomach and large intestine in a clockwise motion and corresponding reflex points on the feet and hands. You can also apply to acupressure points ST3.

Earth Weakened Blends:
Blend #3, Clary Sage, Rose, Nutmeg, Geranium. Massage on lower abdomen and back for menstrual cramps. Blend #4, Clove, Nutmeg, Ginger. Massage on stomach and lower abdomen for cramps.

Chinese constitutional herbal formula that complements the essential oils for Earth Weakened Wen Zong.

Water

Corresponding meridian and energy channels: kidneys (Yin), bladder (Yang).

WATER STRESSED
Edema, swollen abdomen causing indigestion, diarrhea, swelling, stiffness and pain in hands and feet, inflammation, burning irritation, swelling of the breast, emotionally not able to let go of trouble and resentments. These individuals hold on to the fluids and emotions.

Essential oils help the Water Stressed individual with these benefits:
Distributes and eliminates moisture in the body.
Relieves pain in the joints.
Releases pressure from the abdomen and chest.
Helps with the urinary tract infection.

Water Stressed Single Essential Oils:
Juniper, Cypress, Sweet Thyme, Roman Chamomile, Geranium, Rosemary, Grapefruit, Lemon, Eucalyptus A, B, C, D, M, O, R, Patchouli, Vetiver A, B, C, M, R, Cedarwood, Pine A, B, C, D, M, R, Fennel, Cinnamon, Hyssop O.

Water Stressed Blends:
Blend #2, Juniper, Geranium, Cypress, Sweet Thyme, Rosemary, Grapefruit, and Vetiver B, C, M.

Qu Shi is the chinese constitutional herbal formula that compliments the essential oils for water stressed .

WATER WEAKENED
   Lower back pain, weak legs, impotence, curvature of the spine, incontinence, tiredness, frequent urination, asthma, adrenal exhaustion, anemia and osteoporosis.

Essential oils help strengthen the Water Weakened individual with these benefits:
Strengthens the structural system.
Increases sexual drive.
Helps relieve pain in the spine and legs.
Relief of frequent urination.
Helps release fears.

Kidney Weakened Single Essential Oils:
Clove, Ginger, Frankincense, Bergamot, Cistus, Red Thyme, Sandalwood, Geranium A, C, M, ON, R.

RECIPE TO STRENGTHEN KIDNEY WEAKENED INDIVIDUAL
   5 drops Cistus essential oil
   10 drops Sandalwood essential oil
   15 drops Geranium essential oil
   1 oz massage oil or Solubol™

   Place essential oils in 1 oz. bottle and add massage oil/Solubol™. Roll the bottle back and forth between your hands to blend the oils. Pour a few drops into your hand. Hold the oil a few seconds to warm it before applying it to the weakened area. Massage on lower back and lower abdomen and corresponding reflex points on the feet and hands twice daily. You can also apply to acupressure points K1 and K2.

   Jian Gu is the chinese constitutional herbal formula that compliments the essential oils for water weakened.

Metal

   Corresponding meridians or energy channels: lungs (Yin), large intestine (Yang)

METAL STRESSED

Very aggressive, always have their shields up, ready to fight, congestion, bronchitis, colds, edema, fluid on the lungs, sinus congestion, muscle tension, sore throat, wheezing, tuberculosis, emphysema, chronic mucousy cough and deep held grief.

Essential Oils help reduce the Metal Stressed individual with these benefits:
Stimulates the lymphatic system.
Helps to decongest the lungs and sinuses.
Deepens the breath and strengthens the voice.
Encourages one to overcome deep held grief.

Metal Stressed Single Essential Oils:
Rose, Eucalyptus, Frankincense, Myrrh, Niaouli, Peppermint, Geranium, Rosemary, Lemon, and Orange A, B, C, D, M, O, R, Black Pepper O, Ylang-Ylang, Jasmine A, B, C, M, R, Pine A, B, C, D, M, R

Metal Stressed Blends:
Blend #1, Niaouli, Peppermint, Rosemary, Lemon A, D, I, M (if not asthmatic). Massage on acupressure point LI 4.

Xuan Fei is the chinese constitutional herbal formula that compliments the essential oils for Metal Stressed.

METAL WEAKENED

Weak, thin, especially in the upper body, lacks muscle tone, a feverish feeling, hacking cough, lacks sleep because of chronic coughing excessive perspiration due to feverish conditions, chronic problems of lungs and sinuses, fatigue and prostate swelling.

Essential oils help Metal Weakened individual with these benefits:
Rids lungs of infections and viruses.
Reduces feverish feeling.
Builds and protects the lung tissue.
Helps one to stand up for himself.
Relieves bronchial spasms, dry cough, hacking, and wheezing.

Metal Weakened Single Essential Oils:
Frankincense, Cypress, Bergamot, Niaouli, Peppermint, Ginger, Orange, Lemon A, B, C, D, I, M, O, ON, R, Lemongrass, Basil, Hyssop, Red Thyme, Fennel O, Clove D, M, O, Lavender A, B, C, D, I, M, ON.

Metal Weakened Blends:
Blend #1, Niaouli, Rosemary, Peppermint, Geranium A, B, C, D, I, M, O, ON, R, Blend #6, Tea Tree, Ravensara, Lavender, Roman Chamomile A, B, C, D, I, M, O, ON, R. Massage on acupressure point L1.

DIFFUSER RECIPE FOR DRY, HARD COUGH/METAL WEAKENED INDIVIDUAL
    10 drops Pine essential oil
    10 drops Clove essential oil
    5 drops Lemon essential oil

Place 25 drops in diffuser. Diffuse 10 minutes three times daily.

Fu Lei is the chinese constitutional herbal formula that compliments the essential oils for metal weakened.

Wood

Corresponding meridians or energy channels: liver (Yin), gall bladder (Yang).

WOOD STRESSED
Anger, resentment, bitterness, neck and shoulder tension, constipation, poor digestion, eye disorders, abdominal pain, menstrual disorders, headaches, migraines, sore throats and fever.

Essential oils help the Wood Stressed individual with these benefits:
Helps with emotional tension, pains, and digestion.
Relieves aches and pains.
Calms the nerves and circulates energy, increases warmth in the body.
Help the person to feel more harmonious with themselves.

Wood Stressed Single Essential Oils:
Roman Chamomile, Ginger, Orange, Lemon, Rose, Geranium,
   Bergamot, Grapefruit A, B, C, D, M, O, ON, R, Cinnamon A, M, O,
   R, Lavender A, B, C, D, M, ON, R.

Wood Stressed Blends:
Blend #7 Rose, Roman Chamomile, Mandarin, Orange, Lavender A, B,
   C, D, M, ON, R.

This is the chinese constitutional herbal formula that compliments the
essential oils for wood stressed.

WOOD WEAKENED
   Anemia, P.M.S, low immune system, agitation, environmental challenges, poor bowel elimination, allergies, fatigue, mood swings and
hypochondria.

Essential oils help the Wood Weakened individual with these benefits:
Balances hormones.
Enhances immunity.
Stimulates the blood and promotes proper circulation.
Soothes the mind.

Wood Weakened Single Essential Oils:
Ginger, Geranium, Rose, Clove, Sweet Thyme, Rosemary, Lemon, Tea
   Tree, Ravensara A, B, C, D, M, O, ON, R, Red Thyme, Fennel,
   Hyssop, Lemongrass O, Cistus, Frankincense, Myrrh, Ylang-Ylang A,
   B, C, D, M, ON, R.

Wood Weakened Blends:
Blend #6 Tea Tree, Ravensara, Roman Chamomile, and Lavender A, B,
   C, D, M, O, ON, R.

Bu Xue is the chinese constitutional herbal formula that compliments
the essential oils for wood weakened .

Heat

Corresponding meridians or energy channels: lymphatic or fluids.

HEAT STRESSED
Inflammation, skin eruptions, headache, hepatitis, flu, colds with fever, insomnia, menopause, endometris, P.M.S. pain, sore throat, dry eyes, irritation of eyes, night sweat and toxic blood.

Essential oils help the Heat Stressed individual with these benefits:
Relieves pain.
Calms and soothes inflamed tissues.
Cleanses the blood.
Rids the body of infection.
Stimulates the flow of urine.

Heat Stressed Single Essential Oils:
Helichrysum, Niaouli, Roman Chamomile, Lavender, Tea Tree, Juniper, Ravensara, Grapefruit, Lemon, Orange, Sweet Thyme, Geranium, Sweet Marjoram A, B, C, M, O, ON, R, Lemongrass O.

Heat Stressed Blends:

This formula helps to detox the body:
Blend #2, Juniper, Cypress, Grapefruit, Vetiver, Sweet Thyme, Geranium A, B, C, M, ON, R.

This formula helps to build the immune system and reduce inflammation:
Blend #6, Ravensara, Tea Tree, Roman Chamomile, Lavender A, B, C, M, O, ON, R.

Quing Re is the chinese constitutional herbal formula that compliments the essential oils for Heat Stressed.

HEAT WEAKENED
Dry, hot hands and feet, dry, flaky skin, thirst, sugar cravings, low blood pressure, fatigue, adrenal exhaustion, P.M.S, menopause, night

sweats, insomnia, memory lapse, blurry vision and constipation. This type needs moist heat to be balanced.

Essential oils that strengthen the Heat Weakened individual with these benefits:
Soothes inflammation.
Balances hormones.
Moistens the body tissues and glands.
Increases circulation.

Heat Weakened Single Essential Oils:
Rose, Geranium, Fennel, Clary Sage A, B, C, D, M, O, ON, R, Jasmine, Ylang Ylang, Sandalwood A, B, C, M, ON, R, Cistus A, B, C, D, M, ON, R

Heat Weakened Blends:
Blend #8, Jasmine, Rose, Ylang Ylang, Sandalwood A, B, C, M, ON, R.

Bu Yin is the chinese constitutional herbal formula that compliments the essential oils for heat weakened .

Energy

ENERGY STRESSED
Abdominal bloating and pain, cold hands and feet, depression, headache, melancholy, inner tension, insomnia, fear, loose stools, lung congestion, morning sickness, P.M.S, menopause, postpartum depression, asthma and anxiety.

Essential oils help the Energy Stressed individual with these benefits:
Builds female reproductive system.
Unlocks mucous in the respiratory system.
Supports the nervous system.
4 Helps with aches and pains.

Energy Stressed Single Essential Oils:
Geranium, Clary Sage, Rose, Cinnamon, Lemon, Bergamot, Orange,

Jasmine, Grapefruit A, B, C, D, M, O, ON, R, Cinnamon O, Jasmine, Patchouli A, B, C, M, ON, R.

Energy Stressed Blends:
Blend #3, Clary Sage, Rose, Nutmeg, Geranium A, B, C, D, M, ON, R, Blend #7, Roman Chamomile, Geranium, Rose, Mandarin, Orange A, B, C, D, M, ON, R, Blend #10, Roman Chamomile, Geranium, Neroli, Rose, Bergamot A, B, C, D, M, ON, R.

Jie Yu is the chinese constitutional herbal formula that compliments the essential oils for Energy Stressed.

ENERGY WEAKENED
Poor immune response, degenerate diseases, extreme fatigue, damage caused to the body by radiation, drugs, surgery, injury, or emotional stress.

Essential oils help the Energy Weakened individual with these benefits:
Builds the immune system.
Decreases severe fatigue.
Rebuilds deteriorating tissues or organs.

Energy Weakened Single Essential Oils:
Helichrysum, Geranium, Peppermint, Tea Tree, Ravensara, Sweet Thyme, Lemon, Grapefruit, Orange, Neroli, Bergamot, Roman Chamomile A, B, C, M, O, ON, R, Clove, Pine, Cinnamon, Red Thyme A, D, M, O, ON, R, Lavender, Bois de Rose A, D, M, ON, R.

Energy Weakened Blends:
Blend #6 Tea Tree, Ravensara, Roman Chamomile, Lavender A, B, C, D, I, M, O, ON, R.

Sheng Mai is the chinese constitutional herbal formula that compliments the essential oils for energy weakened.

Bibliography

Dharmananda ,S, Ph.D., *Your Nature, Your Health: Chinese Herbs in Constitutional Therapy*, Institute for Traditional Medicine and Preventive Health Care,1986.

Kaptchuk, Ted. *The Web Has No Weaver: Understanding Chinese Medicine,* Congdon & Weed, 1983.

Kaminski ,Patricia, Katz, Richard. *Flower Essence Repertory.* The Flower Essence Society, 1996.

Ritchason, Jack. *The Little Herb Encyclopedia.* 3rd ed., Woodland Health Books, 1994.

Valnet, Jean, *The Practice of Aromatherapy.* Healing Arts Press, 1990.

To learn more about Aromatherapy

Jardin de la Terre
34192 7th Standard Road
Bakersfield, CA 93312
classes, certification, and essential oils

Aromatherapy Institute and Research
P.O. Box 2354
Fair Oaks, CA 95628
certification courses

Journals

Aromatic Thymes
75 Lakeview Parkway
Barrington, IL 60010

Associations

National Associations of Holistic Aromatherapy
P.O. Box 17622
Boulder, CO 80308

The Herb Research Foundation
1007 Pearl Street,Ste.200
Boulder, CO 80302

The Flower Essence Society
P.O. Box 459
Nevada City, CA 95959

Index

sunburn 61, 73, 84, 140

sweet marjoram 28, 38, 43, 95, 112, 116–118, 121–124, 126–129, 131, 133–134, 137–138, 142, 157, 159, 166

sweet thyme 17, 20, 27, 33, 35, 40, 57, 83, 85–86, 95–96, 102, 113, 115–116, 118–119, 121, 128–135, 137–140, 142, 161, 165–166, 168

taste 92

tea tree 17, 22–23, 26, 30–32, 34–35, 45, 49, 60, 74, 79, 85–87, 95, 97–98, 106, 117–119, 123, 125, 128–132, 134–135, 137–140, 164–166, 168

teething 57, 89, 136

temper tantrums 60

tension 12, 19, 24, 41, 49, 51, 54, 63, 65, 68, 72–73, 78, 94, 103–104, 109–111, 123, 125, 127, 129–130, 163–164, 167

tension releaser recipe 41

tiredness 48–49, 68, 98, 105, 110, 125, 129–130, 162

tongue 37, 65, 140

toning 16, 47, 50–52, 55, 58, 64, 67, 70–71, 81, 85, 99, 102, 110, 113, 127, 132, 139–140

toothache 18, 57, 80, 136, 140

touch 7, 92, 111

trauma 53, 73, 156

tuberculosis 56, 60–61, 69–70, 73–74, 79, 83–85, 87–88, 119, 134, 163

uplifting 88, 93, 110, 125–126

urinary system 5–6, 49, 52–53, 57–59, 61, 63–64, 67, 72, 74–75, 80, 82–84, 86, 88–89, 92, 94, 96–97, 102, 142

uterine bleeding 63

uterine cancer 65, 132

uterus 50, 55, 57, 65, 90, 103, 109, 132

vaginal bleeding 65

vaginal discharge 69, 132

vaginitis 51, 73, 77–78, 88–90, 96, 98, 132

varicose veins 58, 64, 74, 83, 91, 113

vertigo 73, 129

viral hepatitis 86, 119

vomiting 66, 74, 82–83, 116

water 11, 19–30, 35–36, 39, 41, 43–50, 54–72, 74–76, 78–97, 102–103, 106–111, 113–114, 118, 122, 136, 141, 143, 156, 161–162

water retention 74–75, 113, 122, 143

weakened 25, 55, 125, 156–168

whooping cough 47–48, 53, 55, 58, 73, 79, 87–88, 91, 97, 101, 119, 134

wood 12–13, 26, 51, 113, 156, 164–165

wrinkles 25, 51, 55, 64, 75, 140

yang 156–157, 159, 161–162, 164

yeast infection 120, 132

yin 156–157, 159, 161–162, 164, 167